EXERCISE AND THE HEART

Guidelines for Exercise Programs

GREATER BOSTON CHAPTER
MASSACHUSETTS HEART ASSOCIATION

Second Printing

EXERCISE

AND THE

HEART

Guidelines for Exercise Programs

Compiled and Edited by

ROBERT L. MORSE, M.D.
Assistant Chief of Medicine
Veterans Administration Hospital
West Roxbury, Massachusetts

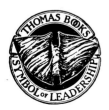

CHARLES C THOMAS · PUBLISHER
Springfield · Illinois · U.S.A.

Published and Distributed Throughout the World by
CHARLES C THOMAS • PUBLISHER
BANNERSTONE HOUSE
301-327 East Lawrence Avenue, Springfield, Illinois, U.S.A.

© *1972, by* CHARLES C THOMAS • PUBLISHER
ISBN 0-398-02365-4
Library of Congress Catalog Card Number: 77-165892

First Printing, 1972
Second Printing, 1974

With THOMAS BOOKS *careful attention is given to all details of manufacturing and design. It is the Publisher's desire to present books that are satisfactory as to their physical qualities and artistic possibilities and appropriate for their particular use.* THOMAS BOOKS *will be true to those laws of quality that assure a good name and good will.*

Printed in the United States of America
00-2

CONTRIBUTORS

Per-Olof Åstrand, M.D.

Department of Physiology—G.I.H.
Fysiologiska Institutionen
Stockholm, Sweden

Carleton B. Chapman, M.D.

Dean, Dartmouth Medical School
Hanover, New Hampshire

William C. Day

Consultant, Physical Fitness
New England Area Council of YMCA's
Kent State University
Kent, Ohio

Stacy H. Dobrzensky, Esq.

Legislative Advisory Committee
American Heart Assiciation
Oakland, California

Lawrence A. Golding, Ph.D.

Director, Applied Physiology Research Laboratory
Kent State University
Kent, Ohio

Burt B. Hamrell, M.D.

Department of Physiology
University of Vermont
Burlington, Vermont

Eugene Z. Hirsch, M.D.

Assistant Professor of Medicine
Case-Western Reserve University
Cleveland, Ohio

William B. Kannel, M.D.

Medical Director
National Heart Institute
Heart Disease Epidemiology Study
Framingham, Massachusetts

Howard G. Knuttgen, Ph.D.

Associate Professor of Physiology
College of Allied Health Professions
and Department of Biology
Boston University
Boston, Massachusetts

Bernard Lown, M.D.

Associate Professor of Cardiology
in Public Health
Harvard School of Public Health
Boston, Massachusetts

Loring B. Rowell, Ph.D.

School of Medicine
Division of Cardiology
University of Washington
Seattle, Washington

FACULTY AND PROGRAM COMMITTEE

FACULTY

Per-Olof Åstrand, M.D.

Grafton Burke, M.D.
Chief of Rehabilitation Services
Josiah B. Thomas Hospital
Peabody, Massachusetts
Professor, School of Allied Health Services
Northeastern University
Boston, Massachusetts

Carleton B. Chapman, M.D.

William C. Day

Stacy H. Dobrzensky, Esq.

Stephen E. Epstein, M.D.
Acting Chief, Cardiology Branch
National Heart Institute
Bethesda, Maryland

Lawrence A. Golding, Ph.D.

Burt B. Hamrell, M.D.

Herman K. Hellerstein, M.D.
Associate Professor of Medicine
Case-Western Reserve University
University Hospital
Cleveland, Ohio

Eugene Z. Hirsch, M.D.

William B. Kannel, M.D.

Howard G. Knuttgen, Ph.D.

Bernard Lown, M.D.

Robert L. Morse, M.D.

Loring B. Rowell, Ph.D.

Arthur A. Sasahara, M.D.
*Associate Professor of Medicine
Harvard Medical School
Boston, Massachusetts*

Douglas R. Rosing, M.D.
*Cardiology Branch
National Heart Institute
Bethesda, Maryland*

PROGRAM COMMITTEE

Howard Knuttgen, Ph.D., Chairman

Robert L. Morse, M.D., Cochairman

Arthur Sasahara, M.D.
*Chairman, Community Program Council
Greater Boston Chapter
Massachusetts Heart Association*

Grafton Burke, M.D.

Paul Couzelis
*Physical Fitness Director
Cambridge YMCA
Cambridge, Massachusetts*

Leonard Covello
*Associate Area Executive
New England Area Council of YMCA's
Boston, Massachusetts*

William Day

Ralph Goldman, Ph.D., Director
*Military Ergonomics
United States Research Institute of Environmental Medicine
Natick, Massachusetts*

Bernard Howes, D.M.D.
Cochairman, New England Area YMCA
Fitness Committee

William Kannel, M.D.

Nathan Kansky
Logistics Chairman

Francis J. O'Brien, D.M.D.
Cochairman, New England Area YMCA
Fitness Committee

Roger Soule, Ph.D.
Assistant Professor of Health Dynamics
Sargent College of Allied Health Professions
Boston University
Boston, Massachusetts

"HEART" STAFF

Mrs. Charlotte M. Crockett
Program Director, Greater Boston Chapter
Massachusetts Heart Association

Lyle Perry
Executive Director, Greater Boston Chapter
Massachusetts Heart Association

**Exercise and the Heart—
Guidelines For Exercise Programs**

Was designed for use by exercise program directors and therefore, by its very nature, is dedicated to them.

KEYNOTE ADDRESS

O NE MIGHT, if he had several hours and a good deal of self-confidence, entitle a keynote address of this sort "The Cultural and Scientific Aspects of Physical Activity." The reason that such a title might make sense is that sociologic, or cultural, attitudes toward physical activity have had, and still have, a great deal to do with public attitudes toward it and, more subtly, have influenced scientific approaches to it.

The physiologist has little trouble agreeing with a statement made several years ago by Erling Asmussen to the effect that the physiology of physical activity includes almost the whole science of physiology. The use of exercise as a research tool appeared almost at the beginning of modern physiology when it became apparent that resting data provide a most incomplete description of the intact organism. The development of quantitative techniques that were applicable to the human being proceeded slowly at first but were far enough along in the 1850's to permit studies by the English physiologist, Edward Smith, that were far in advance of their time. Smith, rather significantly, did his work on prisoners who had been sentenced to hard labor on the infamous prison treadmill. Under the penal system of the time, physical activity was used to degrade human beings, a fact of which the upper strata of British society did not like to be reminded. In any case, Smith did not, it seems, belong to the right social and scientific groups in Britain, and although he was admitted to the Royal Society, his work was largely ignored until Haldane took it up and extended it, ignoring his contributions entirely, in the latter part of the nineteenth century.

Technologic advances before and after the turn of the century permitted marked advances in our understanding of the organism's response to physical stress and led, just before World War I, to the development of the concept of maximal oxygen intake as a measure of the capacity of the organism to respond to a physical challenge. This was one of the genuine landmarks in the development of

[xiii]

physiological thought and knowledge. That concept, and others that derive from it, brought exercise physiology into a new period with the result that, for a time, it virtually dominated the field.

After the war, the development of the acetylene method for measuring cardiac output, a technique that has now fallen into disuse, permitted a considerable extension of our understanding of the quantitative effects of exercise stress on circulatory function. More recent methods for measuring the same variable have resulted, especially in the hands of our Scandinavian colleagues, in further extension of that knowledge and, together with other technologic developments, have opened the way for detailed studies of the effects of physical conditioning, among many other things.

All this vast work led, down the years, virtually to a rewriting of circulatory and respiratory physiology, and had important implications for metabolism as well. In this connection it is appropriate to mention the far-reaching contributions of the Harvard Fatigue Laboratory, established in 1927, ended in 1946. Had it been able to survive a few more years, until NIH research funds became available, it might well still be in operation. But over the short span of its life, the Fatigue Laboratory had a profound effect on physiology in general, and on exercise and altitude physiology in particular, both in this country and abroad.

Exercise physiology, in our own day, has begun to approach limits, of sorts, insofar as the acute response to physical stress is concerned. There is a great deal yet to be learned about the nature of physical conditioning, about control systems that govern the mammalian response to stress, and about the role of the muscle cell itself in the response of the organism to physical stress. Remaining problems now involve much more than what used to be called classical physiology.

But the field is now taking new turnings and some of these involve sociologic or cultural considerations. In medicine, the diagnostic, curative, and rehabilitative value of exercise is now seldom doubted and rests on solid experimental ground. But the use of exercise as a refined, therapeutic tool, as well as the effects of prolonged activity, are not yet firmly accepted since they run counter to well-entrenched notions about the alleged therapeutic value of bedrest.

Regular, heavy exercise has not always been considered quite respectable in western society. In Britain and the United States, it has traditionally been thought that heavy exercise, especially in the form of participation in competitive sports, was best limited to the younger age groups. A lifetime of physical exercise was thought to be proper only for laborers and not for those who, because of education and social standing, had reached the upper income brackets. In Britain, for example, a still popular expression refers to *laboring like a navvy*, and no one would, for good reason, understand if one spoke of laboring like a Cabinet Minister or a business executive.

A certain price has probably been paid for looking on physcial inactivity beyond the age thirty as an essential feature of good breeding and fiscal success. But the full nature and magnitude of the price remain in some doubt.

Does physical inactivity shorten the life span, and does it predispose to coronary disease? A great deal of work, much of it epidemiologic, suggests that the answer must be yes. Most of us who have been interested in the field are convinced that the answer is indeed yes, but despite this, statisticians and scientific purists not infrequently show us that cause and effect relationships are not firmly established. They accuse us of bias both in designing inquiries and in evaluating data. They are no doubt to some extent correct, but their criticisms do not mean that the various studies done to date are invalid. It is apparent to us all, however, that the nature of the problem is such that a definitive answer, acceptable to everyone, will require decades, not years.

From my own bias, there probably is a positive relationship between physical inactivity, on the one hand, and decreased life expectancy, as well as coronary disease, on the other. Yet I think we are today belaboring both issues. The possibility of a positive relation is important even though final proof may still be lacking. And there are other possibilities which, though unproved, are also important. One is that the human being can continue to be physically active, all his life, if he exercises regularly and vigorously from an early age, instead of living out his final years in bed or in a wheelchair. Another is the tranquillizing effect of physical activity, an effect to which most of us can give personal testimony and one which common sense tells us is usually much more practicable than chemical tranquillization.

But probably even more important is the effect of controlled activity in the diagnosis and rehabilitation of the patient with coronary disease. Qualitatively, the value of physical activity in this regard seems now to be beyond much question. What remains is the important business of defining indications and techniques so that the danger of misuse of an important application of earlier knowledge, deriving from various laboratories, can be avoided.

The field of exercise physiology has thus become a unifying theme, bringing the most basic of scientists into intellectual rapport with the clinical scientist. The sports physician and physiologist is also, after many years of isolation, being admitted to the circle. His exclusion, until relatively recently, was not altogether unjustified, but the doctrinaire and superstitious sports trainer of former years is losing his grip. He is, however, being replaced, especially on the American social scene, by the exploitive faddist who seeks to make millions on exercise clubs and absurdly expensive (and often ineffective) exercise apparatus, taking his start from cynical misuse of the work of some of the men on this program.

Perhaps this sort of thing cannot be prevented. But the fact that it happens suggests an added obligation to take the possibility into account when we are dealing with the press or are sought out with flattering offers by various manufacturers. No mechanical apparatus at all, electronic or otherwise, is really essential, provided one has the use of his legs, in availing himself of the benefits of physical activity.

But be all this as it may, exercise physiology is now proceeding in two equally respectable mainstreams: one becomes ever more basic and points increasingly to cellular and subcellular factors; the other brings the body of knowledge that has accumulated since the turn of the century into the lives of individual human beings, with or without established disease. The field as it now stands points out an extremely valuable lesson for the biosciences in general: the basic and the applied scientist are each indispensable and are each rendering a vital public service. The representation of *service*, on the one hand, and *research*, on the other hand as two separate and virtually unrelated entities is, therefore, absurd. And it is even less defensible for the basic scientist to sniff at his colleague who is working on the application of valid scientific findings. This sort of one-upmanship within our own ranks comes as close as anything can to being bio-scientific mortal sin.

The nature of the titles that make up this symposium, and the personalities and insight of the men who have done the work, collectively contrive to show me that everything I have said is redundant. The exercise physiologist has traditionally shown little interest in artificial delineations of what is good and what is not good in science. His ultimate concern has always been for the intact whole organism and all that may affect it. He is now beginning to reap his proper reward, and I count it one of the primary functions of those of us who have turned to executive roles to make it possible for him to keep on with his good work.

CARLETON B. CHAPMAN

PREFACE

ENTHUSIASM FOR becoming "physically fit" has gained great momentum during the past several years. Accordingly, many programs purporting to improve fitness flourished. These included groups of men who, with little or no informed medical supervision, jogged together, lifted weights, performed setting-up exercises, and steamed off a few pounds, reassured that a major factor in the etiology of coronary artery disease was being corrected.

Groups such as the YMCA, on the other hand, long involved in the development of activities to improve fitness, greatly expanded their scope to accommodate the large number of men who sought assistance through an organized program. It became apparent then that existing information concerning many facets of the relationship between exercise and physical fitness was inadequate. In particular, there were no guidelines which could be applicable to a large and heterogeneous population such as those enrolled in many diverse programs in the "Y."

To meet these needs, the Greater Boston Chapter of the Massachusetts Heart Association, in conjunction with the New England Area Council of YMCA's, sponsored this Symposium on Exercise And The Heart at the Sheraton-Boston Hotel, on October 10-11, 1969. Topics designed to answer many of the questions were organized into a coherent program under the direction of Doctors Howard Knuttgen (Chairman) and Robert L. Morse (Cochairman).

It was the primary intent of this symposium to develop practical guidelines for physical fitness programs as well as to make available these guidelines and the original manuscripts to all interested persons.

ARTHUR A. SASAHARA

ACKNOWLEDGMENTS

WE ARE GRATEFUL to William Day and Grafton Burke who proposed the idea of a symposium on exercise as a joint venture of the Greater Boston Chapter of the Massachusetts Heart Association and the YMCA.

Acknowledgments are also due to other members of the Symposium Committee: Paul Couzelis, Leonard Covello, Ralph Goldman, Bernard Howes, Willam Kannel, Nathan Kansky, Francis O'Brien, and Roger Soule.

The symposium was supported in part by grants from the Postgraduate Programs of Merck Sharp and Dohme, Ciba Pharmaceutical Company, Mead Johnson and Company, and Cooper Laboratories, also, the President's Council on Sports and Physical Fitness.

Finally, we would like to make special acknowledgments to the "Heart" staff: Charlotte Crockett, Program Director of the Greater Boston Chapter, who with her staff was responsible for all of the many details necessary to hold a successful symposium, and Lyle Perry, Executive Director of the Chapter, whose total support and guidance were gratefully received throughout this project.

ARTHUR A. SASAHARA
ROBERT L. MORSE

CONTENTS

PART I

SYMPOSIUM ON EXERCISE AND THE HEART

PART II

GUIDELINES FOR EXERCISE PROGRAMS

EXERCISE AND THE HEART

Guidelines for Exercise Programs

PART I

SYMPOSIUM ON EXERCISE AND THE HEART

Chapter 1

HUMAN CARDIOVASCULAR
RESPONSES TO EXERCISE*

LORING B. ROWELL†

Many factors influence the cardiovascular response to muscular exercise. Not only do responses vary with respect to age (16) and sex (2) but also with changes in body posture (gravitational effects) (3, 4, 5, 39). The fraction of the total muscle mass involved at a given level of oxygen uptake (3, 39), environmental factors (31, 32) (heat, altitude, etc.), and state of body hydration (36) are all important modifying factors.

Because of limitations inherent in the scope of any symposium, this presentation focuses upon responses elicited by moving the body mass at controlled rates from one place to another and upon additional cardiovascular adjustments necessitated by prolongation of this task. The discussion is further restricted to responses in normal young men except in cases where appropriate disease models effectively illustrate mechanisms.

Two factors in the total cardiovascular response have been isolated for more detailed description and analysis, namely (a) the role of redistribution of cardiac output with exercise and (b) the importance of competing thermoregulatory demands during work, a possible limiting factor when effort is prolonged. From the former, (a), an attempt is made to illustrate how human cardiovascular responses to work can be scaled and compared in those having wide differences in function and capacity.

---

* Studies from the author's laboratory were supported by National Heart Institute Grant-in-Aid HE-09773 and by the Clinical Research Center facility of the University of Washington, supported by the National Institutes of Health (Grant FR-37) and the Washington State Heart Association.
† Established Investigator of the American Heart Association.

Finally, because of the concern of this symposium with clinical and testing applications, circulatory consequences of carrying out work with small muscle groups, e.g. arms, and of isometric work, will be discussed briefly.

HOW IS OXYGEN TRANSPORT TO WORKING MUSCLES INCREASED, AND WHAT ARE NORMALLY THE LIMITING FACTORS?

The rate of delivery of oxygen from the lungs into the pulmonary capillaries must, of course, increase very drastically. This is primarily accomplished in two ways: (a) by a marked increase in alveolar ventilation and (b) by a redistribution of blood flow within the various regions of the lungs so that all ventilated alveoli become well perfused (44). In normal subjects up to maximal exertion, measurements of arterial oxygen saturation and pO_2 reveal that alveolar ventilation and gas transfer across alveolar membranes to red cells within the pulmonary capillaries are not *normally* limiting factors in total oxygen transport (23, 35).

The major mechanisms by which oxygen transport is augmented are well known. Cardiac output and total oxygen extraction or arteriovenous (A-V) oxygen difference increase. The extent to which they can increase determines the extent to which oxygen transport can increase, that is, they are normally the limiting factors. Work which requires the maximal cardiac output and maximal A-V oxygen difference, by definition, elicits the maximal oxygen consumption. The latter by itself has been shown to represent a sensitive and reproducible measurement (9, 40) of the functional capacity of the cardiovascular system (2, 8, 17, 23, 35). By rearranging terms in the Fick equation, as it is normally expressed, the following statement represents an algebraic expression of this fact.

Maximal oxygen uptake $=$ (maximal heart rate) $\times$ (maximal stroke volume) $\times$ (maximal A-V O_2 difference).

How then is the clinician or physiologist to evaluate the cardiovascular response to exercise? How can different individuals be compared?

To scale anything adequately it is essential to define the full scale response—in this case, the maximal oxygen uptake which defines the full-scale response of the cardiovascular system, i.e. its maximal capacity to transport oxygen to working tissues.

To introduce the concept of scaling and comparing cardiovascular responses to exercise, three types of subjects will be used as examples: (a) endurance athletes, (b) sedentary men, and (c) patients with "pure" mitral stenosis. These patients had essentially normal cardiac outputs and hepatic clearance of indocyanine green dye (thus, normal hepatic blood flow) at rest. None were congested nor in failure (8).

In Figures 1-1 to 1-4, responses of heart rate, stroke volume, their product, cardiac output, and A-V oxygen difference are shown over the full range of oxygen uptake for each group. Values for each are scaled so that body size is eliminated as a factor. The following features are revealed when their responses are compared: (a) The point on the x-axis (oxygen uptake) at which each slope terminates reveals large differences in the magnitudes of maximal oxygen uptake for each group. The slopes relating heart rate (Fig. 1-1) and also A-V oxygen difference (Fig. 1-2) to oxygen uptake, increase to approximately the same maximal values on the y-axis for the three groups. Thus, the slope increases as the maximal oxygen uptake becomes smaller. Differences in stroke volume (Fig. 1-3) reflect the differences in maximal oxygen uptake of the three types of subject, being largest in the athlete and smallest in the patients with mitral stenosis. These differences exist both during supine rest and up to maximal oxygen uptake (4, 5, 8, 17, 22, 35). The dip in stroke volume represents the 40-50 percent fall with assumption of upright posture (22, 42). Even very mild exercise quickly restores stroke volume to supine or baseline values (2, 22, 42). There is little or no rise thereafter with increasing oxygen uptake (2, 22, 42). There is possibly a 10 percent increase in endurance athletes at maximal oxygen uptake; however, data is not sufficient to attach statistical significance to this increment (2, 22). Finally, the increases in cardiac output over the full range of response (Fig. 1-4) reveal that, up to a point, higher heart rate compensates for lower stroke volume in the sedentary man. But at maximal oxygen uptake and maximal heart rate (which is similar in sedentary men and athletes), the lower maximal cardiac output reflects the lower stroke volume of the sedentary

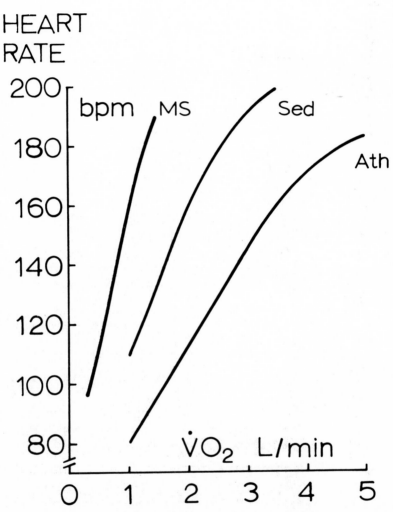

Figure 1-1. The relationship between heart rate and oxygen uptake in athletes (ath), sedentary young men (sed), and patients with pure mitral stenosis (MS) (8, 33). Slopes terminate at the maximal oxygen uptake of each group (5.2, 3.5, and 1.6 liters/min).

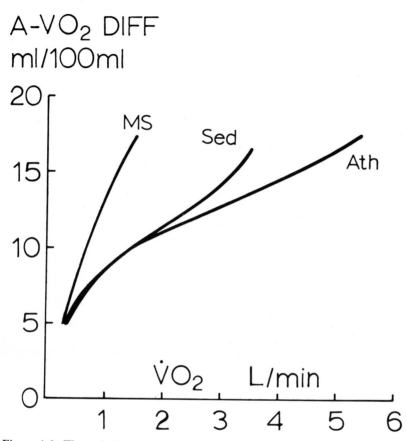

Figure 1-2. The relationship between arteriovenous (A-V) oxygen difference and oxygen uptake up to maximial oxygen uptake in three groups—as coded in Figure 1-1 (2-5, 22, 25, 37, 42).

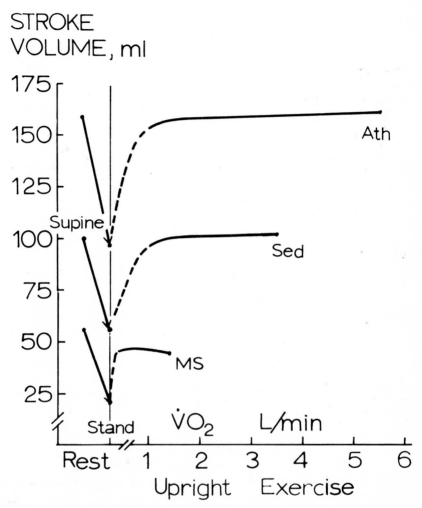

Figure 1-3. The relationship between stroke volume and oxygen uptake in the three groups. On the left is shown the change from supine rest to standing rest—at the vertical line. Note the slight tendency for stroke volume to rise in athletes (ath) and fall in patients with mitral stenosis (MS). Dashed lines indicate the reversal of gravitational effects on stroke volume as exercise begins. This increase may be much more sudden at the onset of upright exercise (22, 42) than for bicycle exercise (2). Data are summarized from (2-5, 22, 25, 37, 42).

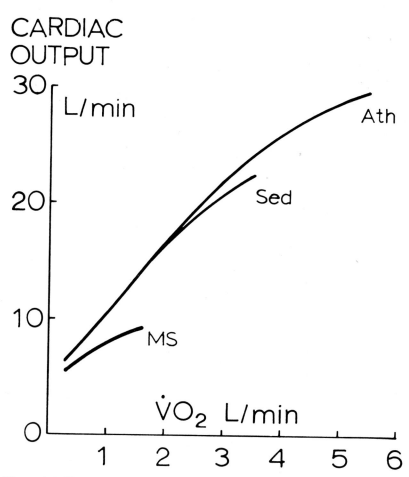

Figure 1-4. The relationship between cardiac output and oxygen uptake in the three groups of individuals (2-5, 22, 25, 31, 37, 42). There is disagreement as to whether cardiac outputs and A-V oxygen differences are the same in athletes and sedentary men at submaximal levels of oxygen uptake 4, 25).

subject. The stroke volumes of the mitral stenosis patients were so low that cardiac output never reached normal values at any level of exercise—despite much higher heart rates (8).

The magnitudes of maximal increase in oxygen transport are shown for the three groups in Table 1-I. The mode of expression in Table 1-I reveals that a major difference between the athlete and his sedentary counterpart is the capacity of the former to raise his heart rate from much lower values at rest (sometimes below 40 beats/min) up to normal maximal levels (190-195 beats/min). The low resting heart rate goes along with his much greater stroke volume. The low stroke volumes of the patients with mitral stenosis give, then, less heart rate reserve. They maintain higher rates at rest and thus have a smaller percentage increase to reach even normal maximal heart rates, as some but not all can do (8). Thus, the major difference in the range of full-scale response of circulatory variables in the three groups was the degree to which heart rate could be increased. Viewed another way, differences in maximal responses are related to the degree to which normal cardiac output at rest is maintained by high heart rate (mitral stenosis) versus high stroke volume and low heart rate (athlete). Heart rate reserve might be thought of as being partially used up by low stroke volume at rest.

Figure 1-2 reveals, again, that augmentation of stroke volume contributes little to increments in oxygen uptake. The tendency for stroke volume to fall slightly in the patients did, however, significantly reduce maximal oxygen uptake because of its greater affect in proportion to the changes in other parameters.

Note the similarity of maximal increments in A-V oxygen difference

TABLE 1-I

MAGNITUDES OF MAXIMAL INCREASE IN THE DETERMINANTS OF MAXIMAL OXYGEN TRANSPORT IN THREE GROUPS HAVING HIGH, NORMAL, AND LOW MAXIMAL OXYGEN CONSUMPTIONS

Group	maximal oxygen uptake	=	heart rate	×	stroke volume	×	A-V oxygen difference
	Increments as Multiples of Resting Values						
Athlete	20	=	4.7	×	1.2	×	3.5
Sedentary	12	=	3.5	×	1.0	×	3.5
Mitral stenosis	6	=	2.3	×	0.8	×	3.1

in the three groups. These data and Figure 1-2 reveal that these three types of individual are all able to extract 80 to 85 percent of the oxygen available from blood. To achieve this degree of extraction, a large percentage of the cardiac output must be distributed to working muscle at the expense of blood flow to nonexercising tissues.

The nonexercising regions which would be expected to have major significance in this response would be the hepatic-splanchnic and renal vascular beds. These regions receive about 50 percent of the cardiac output at rest, but extract a relatively small percentage of the available oxygen (41). Thus, their flow can be reduced markedly before limiting their oxygen uptake.

Figure 1-5A reveals the decrements in hepatic-splanchnic blood flow (HBF) with increasing levels of oxygen consumption in the three groups. At a given level of absolute oxygen consumption (liters per minute) those with the lowest maximal oxygen uptakes have the greatest reduction in HBF (8, 26, 27). Grimby (18) has shown a similar response for renal blood flow in normal subjects differing in maximal oxygen uptake capacity.

Thus, increasing demands for oxygen transport to muscle are met by redistributing more and more blood flow from the visceral region. Figure 1-5B reveals that this response is much more closely related to the percent of maximal oxygen uptake required (relative oxygen uptake) in each group than to absolute metabolic rate. Similar relationships were revealed for heart rate and A-V oxygen difference when responses of these patients were similarly compared with normal subjects (8). Accordingly, differences in the cardiovascular responses to given levels of submaximal exercise among these three groups closely reflect differences in the required fractions of their respective maximal oxygen uptakes and/or maximal cardiac outputs. Stroke volume is the exception. Now these subjects' responses have been scaled in a physiologically comparable manner.

By the 80 percent reduction in HBF, which is eventually reached as maximal oxygen uptake is approached, an additional 300 to 400 ml of O_2 per minute can be made available to working muscle. A similar magnitude of response by the renal circulation would add an additional 200 to 300 ml of oxygen. Thus, redistribution of left ventricular output can supply an additional 500 to 600 ml of oxygen

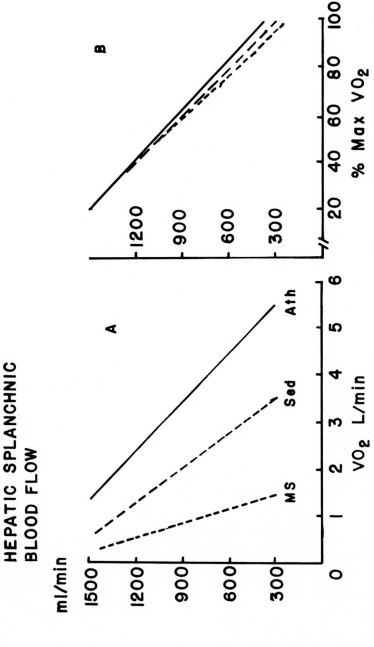

Figure 1-5. The relationship between splanchnic blood flow and absolute oxygen uptake (A) and relative oxygen uptake (percent of maximal) (B) in the three groups. At any given submaximal level of oxygen uptake the reduction in visceral blood flow is inversely proportional to the maximal oxygen uptake or maximal cardiac output (8, 26, 27).

to muscle each minute without requiring additional cardiac output. Additional, smaller quantities are also redistributed away from nonworking muscle and probably other nonworking tissues as well (11, 28, 37, 41).

The quantitative significance of this redistribution of blood flow is inversely related to the magnitude of maximal oxygen uptake. That is, in the athlete who can consume 5 to 6 liters of O_2 per minute (1, 33, 34), this redistribution can account for only about 10 percent of the total oxygen uptake. In the sedentary man it can account for about 20 percent of the total. In the patients with pure mitral stenosis this redistribution can account for approximately 40 percent of total oxygen uptake during maximal work. Now if we challenge with mild exercise a functional Class III or IV (criteria of the New York Heart Association) cardiac patient with essentially fixed cardiac output, 100 percent of the increased demand for oxygen must be met in this way (41). Thus, as the functional capacity of the cardiovascular system decreases from one type of individual to another, an increasingly larger fraction of total oxygen uptake depends upon redistribution of blood flow away from nonworking tissues.

If we now reexamine the three groups on an absolute scale, we see again similar maximal heart rates and maximal A-V oxygen difference (Table 1-II). Their circulatory mechanisms of reaching maximal oxygen uptake are very similar. Stroke volume is the determinant of oxygen transport which most obviously separates the three groups. In the examples chosen, it is the primary factor responsible for the large differences in total oxygen transport. Briefly, other clinical illustrations here would be, for example, those who are limited by heart rate response (heart block). Others can be

TABLE 1-II

MAXIMAL VALUES OF CIRCULATORY DETERMINANTS OF MAXIMAL OXYGEN UPTAKE IN THREE TYPES OF INDIVIDUAL

			Maximal				
Group	oxygen uptake	=	heart rate	×	stroke volume	×	A-V oxygen difference
Athlete	5,200	=	190	×	160	×	17/100
Sedentary	3,500	=	200	×	110	×	16/100
Mitral stenosis	1,600	=	190	×	50	×	17/100

limited by low maximal A-V oxygen difference caused by uneconomical distribution of cardiac output with too large a fraction perfusing nonexercising regions (vasoregulatory asthenia) (21) or by reduced hemoglobin content (38) and so on.

The responses described above are achieved through active, reflex changes in resistance vessels (arterioles) supplying the visceral organs. These responses may serve another crucial role. Despite massive vasodilatation in working muscle, mean arterial blood pressure is well maintained (20, 28). One might view visceral vasoconstriction as an adjunct to increased cardiac output for counter-balancing muscle vasodilatation. Resistances of the system appear to be well balanced. From rest to maximal exercise aortic mean pressure rises only about 20 mm Hg (28).

It is important to point out here that resistances are not so well balanced when work is carried out with small rather than large muscle groups, for example, in work with the arms (3, 39). Very briefly, with arm work as opposed to leg work at the same oxygen uptake we have the following: (a) higher heart rate, (b) lower stroke volume, (c) lower cardiac output, and (d) higher A-V oxygen difference (3, 39). Peripheral vascular resistance and arterial blood pressure are much higher (3, 39). Clearly, these responses reflect greater cardiovascular "strain." It appears as though reflex vasoconstriction in all nonworking regions is still related to the level of oxygen uptake, but because of the decreased ratio of active, vasodilated tissue mass to inactive vasoconstricted tissue mass, pressure and resistance increase. Also, the reflexes driving heart rate and cardiac output appear excessive for the relatively small degree of vasodilatation. Clearly, the increase in cardiac output is not properly compensated for by an appropriate level of vasodilatation or lack of vasoconstriction.

Lind and McNicol (24) have shown this situation to be even more pronounced when work with the arms is isometric. Here the most striking cardiovascular response is severe hypertension. Mean pressure may rise 60 mm Hg during an isometric grip at 50 percent of maximal voluntary contraction force. Clearly this form of exercise is strongly contraindicated in the cardiac patient.

Thus, the two types of arm work briefly described reveal a relatively "excessive" reaction of resistance vessels within unidentified regions.

Returning again to less stressful forms of exercise, in addition to the compensatory adjustments in the resistance vessels, there are equally important adjustments in the peripheral venous bed, i.e. the capacitance vessels, in response to exercise (6, 7, 19, 37). As cardiac output increases with increasing severity of exercise, peripheral venous tone increases proportionally (6, 7, 19). This decrease in venous compliance or "stiffening" of the peripheral venous bed reduces the time constant of the capacitance system. Thus, with vasodilatation of working muscle, blood is rapidly redistributed from peripheral veins and returned without delay or pooling to the central circulation. In this way central venous pressure and volume and ventricular filling pressure and stroke volume are all maintained up to maximal heart rate and maximal cardiac output. In short, these active changes in the peripheral venous bed prevent lags in venous return and shift blood from the periphery to the central vasculature. This response forms a major focal point for the discussion of mechanisms for maintaining oxygen transport which follows.

HOW IS OXYGEN TRANSPORT MAINTAINED WHEN EXERTION IS PROLONGED?

Now the cardiovascular system is confronted with a dual challenge: (a) continued supply of oxygen to working skeletal muscle and vital organs, (b) supplying cutaneous blood flow adequate for conduction of heat from deep tissues to the body surface.

In attacking this problem it will be helpful to visualize some arbitrary shape of the vascular container under normal resting conditions and how the shape of this container may change under the stresses described below (Fig. 1-6). In the early moments of exercise its shape changes. That is, blood volume shifts via reflex venoconstriction from capacious skin (6, 7), and presumably from visceral venous beds as well, to the central vasculature. Resistance vessels of the viscera and nonworking muscle constrict. Resistance vessels in working muscles dilate. In short, blood volume and blood flow may be visualized as being concentrated within major central vessels and the vasculature of working muscle.

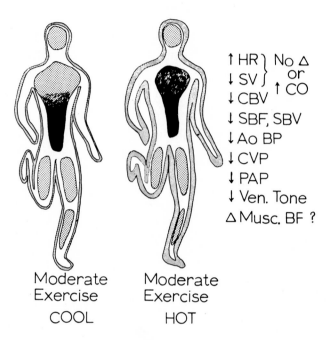

Moderate
Exercise
COOL

Moderate
Exercise
HOT

Figure 1-6. Schematic representation of changes in the shape of the vascular container with upright exercise in a cool environment (left) and exercise in a hot environment (right). Darkened areas reveal sites where flow and/or volume have been reduced.

With exercise (cool) pulmonary volume, the upper portion of the trunk region is restored to that seen in supine rest (lightly shaded region), whereas blood flow and volume of the lower, visceral portion of the trunk (darker region) is reduced (26, 27). There is increased volume and flow of blood in the skin (shaded portion, surrounding the body) and working muscle of the legs.

With exercise in a hot environment, pulmonary blood volume falls (31, 32) along with further reduction in visceral blood flow and volume (27). Skin blood flow and volume are markedly increased. Symbols on the right represent the major cardiovascular changes when heat and exercise stresses are superimposed. From top to bottom the symbols indicate the following: increased heart rate and decreased stroke volume with no change in or increased cardiac output; *decreased* central blood volume, splanchnic blood flow and volume, aortic mean pressure, central venous pressure, pulmonary arterial pressure and venous tone; changes in muscle blood flow are still undefined.

With heat stress superimposed on the metabolic stress of exercise, this distribution of vascular volume, which is optimized for exercise alone, changes again (Fig. 1-6). Environmental heat stress, if sufficient, will abolish cutaneous venous tone (6, 7, 32). This high capacity system dilates. Blood volume and flow are relocated toward the skin. Blood volume shifts from central to peripheral vessels. Pulmonary blood volume falls (30, 31), and there is further reduction of visceral blood volume and flow (27). Stroke volume is reduced, and cardiac output is maintained by tachycardia (31, 32, 45). Arterial and central venous blood pressure fall, and work capacity is reduced, sometimes drastically (31, 32). This response to exercise in a hot environment is not unlike the cardiovascular response which *gradually* develops during prolonged moderate to heavy exercise in cooler environments.

The studies of Ekelund and Holmgren (12-15) (Fig. 1-7) and also Saltin and Stenberg (36) showed a marked rise in heart rate during prolonged work. Oxygen uptake and A-V oxygen difference also increased but less markedly (less than 10%). Cardiac output remained constant, and total blood volume fell only slightly during the first minutes of work and remained constant thereafter. On the other hand, both systemic and pulmonary arterial pressures and also stroke volume fell continuously throughout the period of prolonged heavy work. A similar downward drift in right ventricular and diastolic pressure as well as a fall in heart volume and central venous pressure were also noted by Ekelund *et al.* (14). Pulmonary blood volume, according to the author, probably fell as well. The rise in oxygen consumption was too small to account for the rise in heart rate. Thus, three major findings characterized the central circulatory response to prolonged heavy exercise: (a) a continuous rise in heart rate, (b) a continuous fall in stroke volume, and (c) a progressive decline in arterial and central venous pressures.

The causes of these changes are not known. Because the drift in these variables was also observed by Ekelund (12) and by Saltin and Stenberg (36) during supine exercise, they argued that the cause was probably changes in the heart, itself, rather than thermally induced dilatation of cutaneous resistance and capacitance vessels, with resultant venous pooling. That is, gravitational pooling of blood

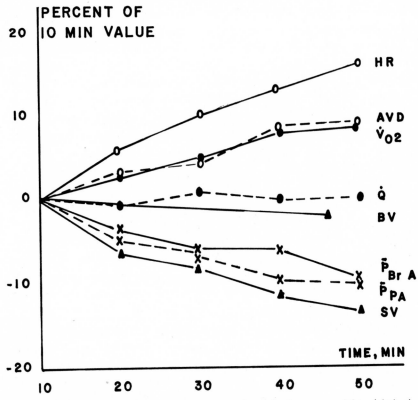

Figure 1-7. Hemodynamic responses to prolonged, heavy upright (sitting) exercise in a cool environment reproduced from published work of Ekeland and Holmgren (15). From top to bottom on the right of the figure, symbols reveal the rises in heart rate, A-V oxygen differences, and oxygen uptake. Cardiac output remained constant. Blood volume fell a few percent during the first ten minutes of exercise. The slight fall shown thereafter was not significant. Decreases in mean brachial and pulmonary arterial pressures and in stroke volume are shown in that order. (Reproduced by permission of the authors and *Acta Physiol Scand*, 62:240-255, 1964.)

in dilated veins was thought to be prevented by supine posture. This point of view is contestable. The relationships between venous compliance, transmural pressure, and surrounding tissue pressure need to be defined. The extent to which increments in cutaneous venous compliance might affect central hemodynamics during supine work has not been investigated. However, these effects have recently been described for prolonged *upright* work (32).

An alternative hypothesis to that of the above workers would be that rising body and skin temperatures are major factors in eliciting these responses. The cardiovascular responses to competitive thermal and exercise stresses, briefly outlined above and in Figure 1-6, suggest such a cause. Recently, all of these changes seen during prolonged exercise were reproduced by suddenly heating a man while he continued to work in the upright posture (32). A water-perfused suit, the undergarment of NASA Apollo suits,* was used to produce sudden, almost square-wave changes in skin temperature. On the other hand, these effects could be reversed by suddenly cooling the sking during exercise, or they could be prevented from occuring at all, as a natural course of events, by maintaining the skin at a low temperature. Accordingly, I wish to propose that a major cause of the drift in these circulatory parameters is a progressive decline in cutaneous venous tone with a peripheral shift in blood volume as well as blood flow to the skin. This is viewed as a reflex thermoregulatory response resulting from the progressive superimposition of thermal stress upon prolonged metabolic stress.

This hypothesis is based on the findings of Bevegård and Shepherd (6, 7) who found that heating a limb abolished its normal venoconstriction or responses to exercise in a manner similar to that seen in the sympatheticized limb (7). Webb-Peploe and Shepherd (43) also found that venous tone was inversely proportional to the temperature of blood perfusing the veins of dogs. A gradual increase in the volume of the capacious cutaneous venous bed would necessitate a shift of blood volume from central vessels. Were blood to accumulate gradually in peripheral veins, venous return would gradually diminish in the absence of compensatory mechanisms. Continued balance between right and left ventricular outputs requires a gradual depletion of preventricular sumps (visceral vasculature?). That is, what is gradually pooled in the periphery would, by necessity, require a compensatory reduction in blood volume of other regions to maintain cardiac output. The shape of the vascular container changes gradually from that depicted in the center of Figure 1-6 (cool) to that on the right (hot). Attending these changes is a gradual decline in central venous and cardiac filling pressure and in stroke volume.

---

* Generously loaned by NASA Manned Space Craft Center, Houston, Texas.

The decline in peripheral vascular resistance which results from gradual vasodilatation of skin is not compensated for by either a rise in cardiac output or sufficient vasoconstriction in nonworking tissues, i.e. arterial pressure falls. Had stroke volume not declined, the rise in heart rate and, thus, in cardiac output would have been sufficient to maintain blood pressure at control levels. In addition to the major causal role proposed for the peripheral venous system, direct thermal effects upon the myocardium could sometimes be involved also. Contractile force of the myocardium may decline when its temperature rises. However, the time trends described above still continue even after right atrial temperature stabilizes (32).

It is possible that other nonthermal effects may contribute to the decline in pressure, etc., described above. Available evidence indicates that, unlike the response of cutaneous resistance vessels, vasoconstriction is well maintained or may increase in renal (10, 18) and splanchnic (29) vascular beds during work. However, it is not known whether vasoconstriction of nonworking muscle persists during prolonged exercise. A gradual decline in the resistance of working muscle is another possibility (this might be of either direct thermal, local metabolic, or central nervous origin). The peripheral venoconstrictor response to exercise has been observed for work periods extending up to only ten minutes (6, 7, 19). The basic question raised here is whether the sympathetic nervous (i.e. vasoconstrictor) outflow, which is initially regulated in proportion to the relative severity of exercise, is maintained, independent of thermal changes, in all arterial and venous beds beyond ten minutes of work. At this time the major cause of the decline in peripheral vascular resistance does appear to be cutaneous vasodilatation.

In conclusion, the major cardiovascular responses to a sudden demand for increased O_2 transport are increased heart rate, cardiac output, and O_2 extraction with little or no change in stroke volume once the response to postural (gravitational) effects is complete. In normal subjects, cardiac output is predictably related to absolute oxygen uptake, up to about 70 percent of the maximal value; heart rate increases, and blood flow to nonworking tissue decreases in proportion to the percent of maximal oxygen uptake required. In normal men, differences in maximal oxygen consumption are due primarily to differences in stroke volume.

The major changes in the cardiovascular system during prolonged work appear to be as follows: (a) Peripheral cutaneous venous tone, which normally increases in proportion to the severity of work, gradually declines, so that blood shifts from the central to peripheral vasculature. (b) Cutaneous vascular resistance also decreases. (c) Cardiac filling pressure, central blood volume, and stroke volume are reduced so that cardiac output must be maintained by tachycardia. (d) The failure of cardiac output to increase while peripheral resistance falls leads to the decline in blood pressure. Redistribution of blood flow and volume toward surface vessels facilitates heat loss. Since the result of the above changes is always increased heart rate, myocardial fatigue could become a factor in limiting work capacity.

REFERENCES

1. Åstrand, P.-O.: New records in human power. *Nature, 176*:922-923, 1955.
2. Åstrand, P.-O., Cuddy, T. E., Saltin, B., and Stenberg, J.: Cardiac output during submaximal and maximal work. *J Appl Physiol, 19*:268-274, 1964.
3. Bevegård, S., Freyschuss, U., and Strandell, T.: Circulatory adaptation to arm and leg exercise in supine and sitting position. *J Appl Physiol, 21*:37-46, 1966.
4. Bevegård, S., Holmgren, A., and Jonsson, B.: Circulatory studies in well trained athletes at rest and during heavy exercise, with special reference to stroke volume and the influence of body position. *Acta Physiol Scand, 57*:26-50, 1963.
5. Bevegård, S., Holmgren, A., and Jonsson, B.: The effect of body position on the circulation at rest and during exercise, with special reference to the influence on the stroke volume. *Acta Physiol Scand, 49*:279-298, 1960.
6. Bevegård, S., and Shepherd, J. T.: Reaction in man of resistance and capacity vessels in forearm and hand to leg exercise. *J Appl Physiol, 21*:123-132, 1966.
7. Bevegård, S., and Shepherd, J. T.: Changes in tone of limb veins during supine exercise. *J Appl Physiol, 20*:1-8, 1965.
8. Blackmon, J. R., Rowell, L. B., Kennedy, J. W., Twiss, R. D., and Conn, R. D.: Physiological significance of maximal oxygen intake in "pure" mitral stenosis. *Circulation, 36*:497-510, 1967.
9. Buskirk, E., and Taylor, H. L.: Maximal oxygen intake and its relation to body composition with special reference to chronic physical activity and obesity. *J Appl Physiol, 11*:72-78, 1957.
10. Chapman, C. B., Henschel, A., Minckler, J., Forsgren, A., and Keys, A.:

The effect of exercise on renal plasma flow in normal male subjects. *J Clin Invest, 27*:639-644, 1948.

11. Donald, K. W., Wormald, P. N., Taylor, S. H., and Bishop, J. M.: Changes in the oxygen content of femoral venous blood and leg blood flow during leg exercise in relation to cardiac output response. *Clin Sci, 16*:567-591, 1957.

12. Ekelund, L.-G.: Circulatory and respiratory adaptation during prolonged exercise in the supine position. *Acta Physiol Scand, 68*:382-396, 1966.

13. Ekelund, L.-G.: Circulatory and respiratory adaptation during prolonged exercise of moderate intensity in the sitting position. *Acta Physiol Scand, 69*:327-340, 1967.

14. Ekelund, L.-G., Holmgren, A., Ovenfors, C. O.: Heart volume during prolonged exercise in the supine and sitting position. *Acta Physiol Scand, 70*:88-98, 1967.

15. Ekelund, L.-G., Holmgren, A.: Circulatory and respiratory adaptation during long-term, non-steady state exercise, in the sitting position. *Acta Physiol Scand, 62*:240-255, 1964.

16. Granath, A., Jonsson, B., Strandell, T.: Circulation in healthy old men, studied by right heart catheterization at rest and during exercise in supine and sitting position. *Acta Med Scand, 176*:425-446, 1964.

17. Grande, F., and Taylor, H. L.: Adaptive changes in the heart, vessels, and patterns of control under chronically high loads. In *Handbook of Physiology.* Washington, D. C., American Physiological Society, 1964, Section 2, Vol. 3.

18. Grimby, G.: Renal clearances during prolonged supine exercise at different loads. *J Appl Physiol 20*:1294-1298, 1965.

19. Hanke, D., Schlepper, M., Westermann, K., and Witzleb, E.: Venentonus Haut-und Muskeldurchblutung an Unterarm und Hand bei Beinarbeit. *Pflügers Arch, 309*:115-127, 1969.

20. Holmgren, A.: Circulatory changes during muscular work in man, with special reference to arterial and central venous pressures in the systemic circulation. *Scand J Clin Lab Invest,* Vol. 8, Suppl. 24, 1956.

21. Holmgren, A., Jonsson, B., Levander, M., Linderholm, H., Sjöstrand, T., and Ström, G.: Low physical working capacity in suspected heart cases due to inadequate adjustment of peripheral blood flow (vasoregulatory asthenia). *Acta Med Scand, 158*:413-436, 1957.

22. Marshall, R. J., and Shepherd, J. T.: *Cardiac Function in Health and Disease.* Philadelphia, Saunders, 1968.

23. Mitchell, J. H., Sproule, B. J., and Chapman, C. B.: The physiological meaning of the maximal oxygen intake test. *J Clin Invest, 37*:538-547, 1958.

24. Lind, A. R., and McNicol, G. W.: Local and central circulatory responses to sustained contractions and the effect of free or restricted arterial inflow on post exercise hyperemia. *J Physiol, (London), 192*:575-593, 1967.

25. Musshoff, K., Reindell, H., and Klepzig, H.: Stroke volume, arteriovenous difference, cardiac output and physical working capacity and their relationship to heart volume. *Acta Cardiol, 14*:427-452, 1959.

26. Rowell, L. B., Blackmon, J. R., Bruce, R. A.: Indocyanine green clearance and estimated hepatic blood flow during mild to maximal exercise in upright man. *J Clin Invest, 43*:1677-1690, 1964.

27. Rowell, L. B., Blackmon, J. R., Martin, R. H., Mazzarella, J. A., and Bruce, R. A.: Hepatic clearance of indocyanine green in man under thermal and exercise stresses. *J Appl Physiol, 20*:384-394, 1965.

28. Rowell, L. B., Brengelmann, G. L., Blackmon, J. R., Bruce, R. A., and Murray, J. A.: Disparities between aortic and peripheral pulse pressures induced by upright exercise and vasomotor changes in man. *Circulation, 37*:954-964, 1968.

29. Rowell, L. B., Kraning II, K. K., Evans, T. O., Kennedy, J. W., Blackmon, J. R., and Kusumi, F.: Splanchnic removal of lactate and pyruvate during prolonged exercise in man. *J Appl Physiol, 21*:1773-1783, 1966.

30. Rowell, L. B., Kraning II, K. K., Kennedy, J. W., and Evans, T. O.: Central circulatory responses to work in dry heat before and after acclimatization. *J Appl Physiol, 22*:509-518, 1967.

31. Rowell, L. B. Marx, H. J., Bruce, R. A., Conn, R. D., and Kusumi, F.: Reductions in cardiac output, central blood volume and stroke volume with thermal stress in normal men during exercise. *J Clin Invest, 45*:1801-1816, 1966.

32. Rowell, L. B., Murray, J. A., Brengelmann, G. L., and Kraning II, K. K.: Human cardiovascular adjustments to rapid changes in skin temperature during exercise. *Circ Res, 24*:711-724, 1969.

33. Rowell, L. B., Taylor, H. L., and Wang, Y.: Limitations to prediction of maximal oxygen intake. *J Appl Physiol, 19*:919-927, 1964.

34. Saltin, B., and Åstrand, P. O.: Maximal oxygen uptake in athletes. *J Appl Physiol, 23*:353-358, 1967.

35. Saltin, B., Blomqvist, G., Mitchell, J. H., Johnson, Jr., R. L., Wildenthal, K., and Chapman, C. B.: Response to submaximal and maximal exercise after bedrest and training. *Circulation,* Vol. 38, Suppl. 7, 1968.

36. Saltin, B., and Stenberg, J.: Circulatory response to prolonged severe exercise. *J Appl Physiol, 19*:833-838, 1964.

37. Shepherd, J. T.: Behavior of resistance and capacity vessels in human limbs during exercise. *Circ Res, 20 (Suppl. 1)*:70-81, 1967.

38. Sproule, B. J., Mitchell, J. H., Miller, W. F.: Cardiopulmonary physiological responses to heavy exercise in patients with anemia. *J Clin Invest, 39*:378-388, 1960.

39. Stenberg, J., Åstrand, P. O., Ekblom, B., Royce, J., and Saltin, B.: Hemodynamic response to work with different muscle groups, sitting and supine. *J Appl Physiol, 22*:61-70, 1967.

40. Taylor, H. L., Buskirk, E., and Henschel, A.: Maximal oxygen intake

as an objective measure of cardio-respiratory performance. *J Appl Physiol, 8*:73-80, 1955.

41. Wade, O. L., and Bishop, J. M.: *Cardiac Output and Regional Blood Flow*. Oxford, Blackwell, 1962.

42. Wang, Y., Marshall, R. J., and Shepherd, J. T.: The effect of changes in posture and of graded exercise on stroke volume in man. *J Clin Invest, 39*:1051-1061, 1960.

43. Webb-Peploe, M. M., and Shepherd, J. T.: Responses of the superficial limb veins of the dog to changes in temperature. *Circ Res, 22*:737-746, 1968.

44. West, J. B.: *Ventilation/Blood Flow and Gas Exchange*. Oxford, Blackwell, 1965.

45. Williams, C. G., Bredel, G. A. G., Wyndham, C. H., Strydom, J., N. B., Morrison, F., Peter, J., Fleming, R. W., and Ward, J. S.: Circulatory and metabolic reactions to work in heat. *J Appl Physiol, 17*:625-638, 1962.

Chapter 2

PHYSIOLOGICAL CONDITION AND ITS ASSESSMENT

PER-OLOF ÅSTRAND

INTERRELATION BETWEEN AEROBIC AND ANAEROBIC ENERGY YIELD

Any engagement in muscular activity demands an extra energy yield above the resting metabolism. Table 2-I gives an approximate summary of the energy content in the body available for muscular work. The figures are subjected to large individual fluctuations, particularly the content of fat. It is assumed that in a well trained man with a body weight of 75 kg, some 20 kg of muscle may be active during running or bicycling.

TABLE 2-I

	Concentration per kg Wet Muscle	Energy/Mole kcal	Total kcal in Man: Body Weight 75 kg, Muscle Weight 20 kg
ATP	6 mM	10	1.2
Creatine phosphate	17 mM	10.5	3.6
Glycogen	15 g	ca. 690	1,200
Fat			50,000

(From various sources; see Åstrand and Rodahl, 1970, p. 19.)

Evidently, the energy supply from the breakdown of the high-energy phosphate compounds would only cover the demand for some seconds of maximal effort. In fact, this may explain why maximal speed can be maintained only for a limited time. The energy yield from glycogenolysis and aerobic processes is a slower process. Quantitively, however, oxygen is the key for unlocking the doors to the great energy stores within the body, and the availability of oxygen to the working muscle cells determines the endurance in prolonged physical work. Figure 2-1 presents an example of efforts to analyze the contribution in the energy yield from aerobic and anaerobic pro-

[27]

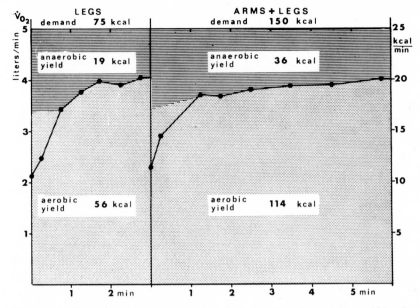

Figure 2-1. Increase in oxygen uptake during exhausting work on bicycle ergometer, following a ten-minute warm-up period. *Left:* illustrates leg work only; *Right:* exercise with the same work load (350 watts) but with both arms (100 watts) and legs (250 watts) involved. Load could be tolerated twice as long with arms and legs working. Calculations of energy demand and yield are explained in text. (From Åstrand and Rodahl, 1970, p. 295. Courtesy of McGraw-Hill Book Publishing Company.)

cesses, respectively. From the work load and the mechanical efficiency of 22 percent for aerobic work on a bicycle the energy demand can be calculated.

During 3 min of exercise, at a rate representing the maximum in leg work for this subject, the energy demand was about 75 kcal. An aerobic energy yield would thus have demanded an oxygen uptake of 15 liters (since 1 liter of oxygen can deliver about 5 kcal in combustion of glycogen). The oxygen uptake was measured continuously and was only 10.7 liters. It is assumed that an additional 0.5 liter was utilized from stores bound to myoglobin and hemoglobin, refilled after the exercise. Therefore the aerobic yield can be estimated to be 56 kcal (11.2×5). The deficit was then $75 - 56 = 19$ kcal, and this energy must have been derived anaerobically. A breakdown of ATP and creatine phosphate may yield 5 to 7.5 kcal, and the remaining deficit of a minimum of about 12 kcal must have been yielded by glycogenolysis and glucolysis with a formation of lactic acid. It can be calculated that for a release of 12 kcal the lactic acid production must be 39 g. With both arms and legs working, the load could be tolerated for 6 min which means an energy output of at least 150 kcal. The measured oxygen uptake of 22.3 liters complemented with 0.5 liter from oxygen stores within the body covers 114 kcal, leaving 36 kcal for the anaerobic processes. The formation of lactic acid must have been of the order of 95 g. The equivalent oxygen deficit was about 6 liters ($=$ 29 kcal). The elimination of 95 g of lactic acid demands, however, 12 liters of oxygen; the oxygen debt therefore will be twice as large as the deficit. In other words, the efficiency of the anaerobic glycogenolysis is about 50 percent of the aerobic breakdown of glycogen. Added should be the so-called alactacid oxygen debt which may be up to 4 liters.

Figure 2-2 shows the relative importance of the aerobic and anaerobic processes in maximal physical efforts of various duration. The calculations are based on the assumption that the individual had a maximal oxygen uptake of 5 liters/min and a maximal anaerobic capacity of 45 kcal. It is also assumed that 100 percent of maximal oxygen uptake can be maintained for ten minutes; 95 percent, for thirty minutes, and eighty-five percent, for sixty minutes. With the exception of athletes' activities, or if one were in a particularly dangerous situation, the anaerobic utilization of glycogen or glucose is in practical life of minor importance. So I will focus the attention on the aerobic power.

AEROBIC POWER

Figure 2-3 illustrates the normal procedure to measure the individual's maximal oxygen uptake, and I also show it to define the term "maximal aerobic power," which is the highest oxygen uptake the individual can attain during physical work breathing air at sea level. To evaluate whether or not the subject's maximal oxygen uptake has been obtained, objective criteria should be used, such as measured oxygen uptake lower than expected from the work load, and blood lactic acid concentration higher than about 8 mM/liter.

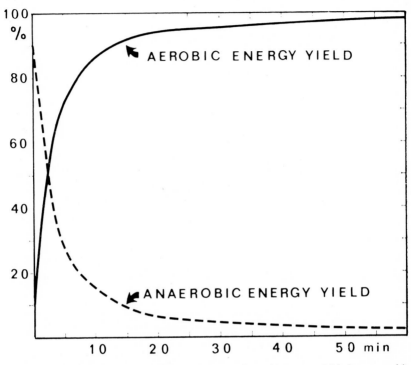

Figure 2-2. Relative contribution in percent of total energy yield from aerobic and anaerobic processes, respectively, during maximal efforts of up to sixty-minutes duration for an individual with high maximal power for both processes. Note that a two-minute maximal effort hits the 50 percent mark, meaning that both processes are equally important for success. (From Åstrand and Rodahl, 1970, p. 304. Courtesy of McGraw-Hill Book Publishing Company.)

A critical question is whether different types of work give the same maximal oxygen uptake. It appears that by running on the treadmill uphill greater than or equal to 3 degrees of inclination the oxygen uptake may be brought to a maximum, while running horizontally or at a slight inclination results in a somewhat lower measured oxygen uptake. Bicycling produces on the average a lower oxygen uptake, at least compared to running uphill. In studies where objective criteria have been used to determine whether or not the maximal oxygen uptake was reached for the type of work in question, the values for running are on an average 5 to 8 percent higher

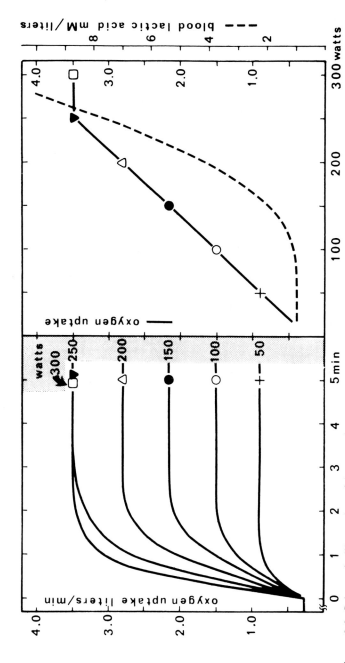

Figure 2-3. Schematic illustration of increase in oxygen uptake during exercise on bicycle ergometer with different work loads (noted within shadowed area) performed during five to six minutes. *To the right*: oxygen uptake in the above-mentioned experiments, measured after five minutes and plotted in relation to work load. Peak lactic acid concentrations in the blood at each experiment are included. On the bicycle ergometer this subject's maximal aerobic power was 3.5 liters/min. (From Åstrand and Rodahl, 1970. Courtesy of McGraw-Hill Book Publishing Company.)

than for bicycling. Thus, Hermansen and Saltin (1969) noticed that in their fifty-five male subjects, 0.28 liter/min (7%) higher oxygen uptake was attained during maximal running compared to bicycling. No significant differences were obtained in maximal values for the work time, pulmonary ventilation, blood lactate, and heart rate (Fig. 2-4). Age or training condition did not seem to influence these results. It is, in a way, unfortunate that the subjects used a pedal frequency of only 50 rpm. As illustrated by Figure 2-5, 60 rpm gave a higher maximal oxygen uptake than did 50 rpm (0.10

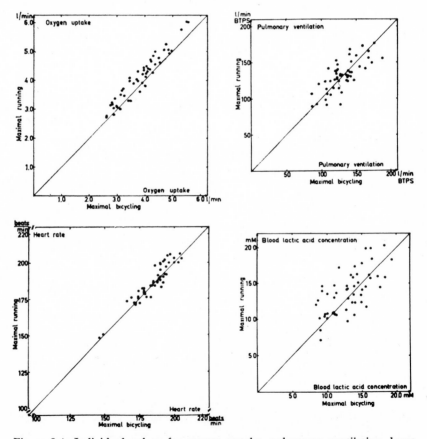

Figure 2-4. Individual values for oxygen uptake, pulmonary ventilation, heart rate, and blood acid concentration during maximal bicycle exercise compared with corresponding values during maximal treadmill exercise. (From Hermansen and Saltin, 1969. Courtesy of *Journal of Applied Physiology.*)

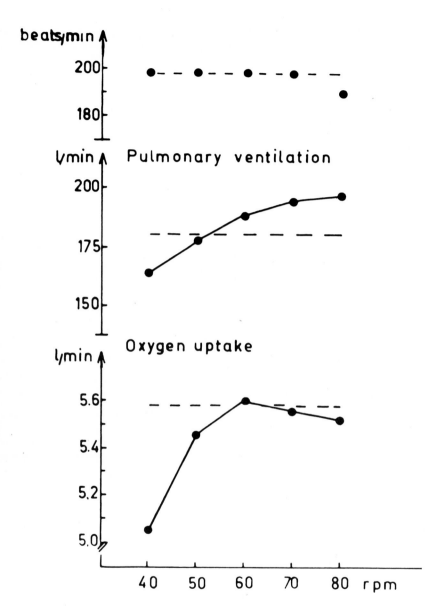

Figure 2-5. Oxygen uptake, pulmonary ventilation, and heart rate during maximal bicycling with different pedal frequences (40-80 rpm) for one subject. For comparison values (*dashed line*) for maximal running up hill (3°) is also included. Work load was in all bicycle experiments 2,700 kpm/min. (From Hermansen and Saltin, 1969. Courtesy of *Journal of Applied Physiology.*)

TABLE 2-II

Study	Number of Subjects	Running Uphill ≥ 3°	Running Horizontal 0 to 1°	Bicycling Legs Sitting	Bicycling Legs Supine	Bicycling Arms and Legs
Åstrand, female	33	...	2.89	2.76		
1952 male	34		4.04	4.03		
Åstrand and Saltin, 1961	5	4.69	...	4.47	3.85	
	6	...	...	4.23	...	4.24
Stenberg et al., 1967	5	...	...	3.87	3.42	3.95
Chase et al., 1966	18	3.86	...	3.28		
Wyndham et al., 1966	40	...	3.08	2.84		
Glassford et al., 1965	24	3.76	...	3.49		
Hermansen	5	4.22	...	4.06		
and Saltin	6	4.68	4.48	4.34		
1969	55	4.16	...	3.90		

liter/min higher for 6 subjects; $p < 0.005$). Table 2-II presents a summary of data obtained on maximal oxygen uptake in different types of exercise. (For complete reference list and discussion see Åstrand and Rodahl, 1970, Chapter 11.)

Hermansen and Saltin (1969) also noted that heart rate, pulmonary ventilation, and blood lactate were somewhat higher on the bicycle compared to treadmill exercise at the same submaximal oxygen uptake. The difference in heart rate was about five and ten beats/min for trained athletes and untrained subjects respectively.

Presently the observed differences in data obtained on treadmill and bicycle ergometer procedures cannot be physiologically explained. To ensure that the highest possible oxygen uptake be attained, the inclination on the treadmill should be 3° or more. For the bicycle test a frequency of 60 up to 70 rpm should be used.

AEROBIC POWER AND PERFORMANCE

It is well established that the individual's maximal oxygen uptake is of decisive importance for his ability to do physical work, not only in his leisure time but also in manual labor. Hansson (1965) noted that lumberjacks with very high earnings were characterized by a particularly high maximal aerobic power, compared to the normal earner. It is also an interesting observation that a worker involved in manual labor, more or less free to set his own pace, normally accepts working with a caloric output which is approximately 40 percent of his aerobic power (I. Åstrand, 1967). In prolonged exercise not only the individual's maximal aerobic power but also the available glycogen stores are of importance for the performance, at least in heavy exercise. With the needle biopsy technique developed by Bergström and Hultman (1966) it is now possible to map out the influence of work and diet on the glycogen content of the muscles. Figure 2-6 presents one example of how the speed for the first hour of a race was independent of the initial glycogen content of the leg muscles, but then speed became eventually reduced depending whether or not glycogen was available. The lower the initial store, the sooner the impairments in running occurred. (See Åstrand and Rodahl, 1970, Chapter 14.)

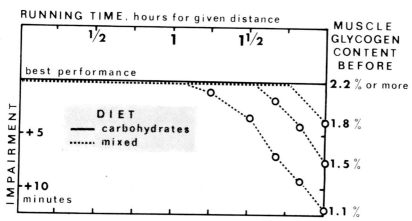

Figure 2-6. Schematic illustration of the importance of a high glycogen content in the muscle before a 30-km race (running). The lower the initial glycogen store, the slower became the speed at the end of the race compared with the race performed when the muscle glycogen content was 2.2 g or higher per 100 g muscle at the start of the race. For the first hour, however, no difference in speed was observed. (By courtesy of Saltin.)

AGE AND SEX

Figures 2-7 and 2-8 give our summary of data on maximal oxygen uptake for women and men of different age. All subjects were healthy and moderately well trained. The women's power is on an

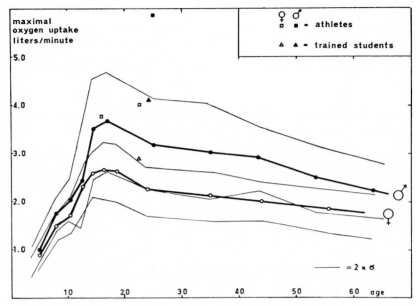

Figure 2-7. Mean values for maximal oxygen uptake (maximal aerobic power) measured during exercise on treadmill or bicycle ergometer in 350 female and male subjects four to sixty-five years of age. Included are values from three athletes and from a group of eighty-six trained students in physical education. (From Åstrand and Christansen, 1964. Courtesy of Pergamon Publishing Company.)

average 70 to 75 percent of that of men. In both sexes there is a peak at eighteen to twenty years of age, followed by a gradual decline in the maximal oxygen uptake. The individual variation should be noticed. Many old subjects had a maximal power that was higher than that found in many much younger individuals. In Figure 2-7 the " −2 standard deviation line" for male subjects coincides closely with the average values for women, and the 95 percent range is actually ± 20 to 30 percent of the mean value at a given age. Since training will in most cases increase the maximal oxygen uptake not more than 10 to 20 percent, it is evident that the natural endowment is the most important factor determining the individual's maximal aerobic power. In other words, the figure for maximal oxygen uptake does not in itself reveal whether or not an individual has been physically active in the preceding years. Gunder Hägg

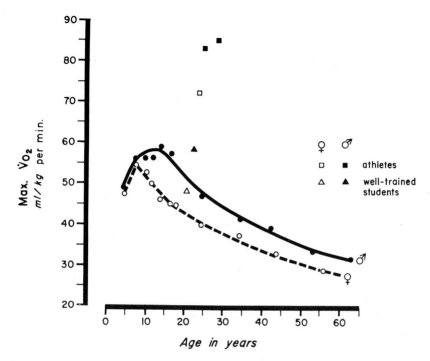

Figure 2-8. Same studies as Figure 2-7, but the maximal $\dot{V}_{O_2}$ is calculated per kilogram of body weight. (From Åstrand and Rodahl, 1970. Courtesy of McGraw-Hill Publishing Company.)

held many world records in middle and long-distance running in the 1940's. He stopped his training in 1946, and when we studied him in 1963, he was completely untrained. However, his maximal oxygen uptake was very high or 4.0 liters/min (age 45 yrs).

In several athletes who competed in endurance events we have found maximal oxygen uptakes exceeding 6.0 liters/min, which is about twice as high as that of the average man.

There are similar data as presented in Figures 2-7 and 2-8 from other countries. The absolute values for maximal oxygen uptake will inevitably vary for different groups and populations; the selection of subjects is rather critical in this respect. The variations observed with age and sex agree, however, with the data in Figures 2-7 and 2-8.

It is well established that the maximal heart rate decreases with

age, from about 210 beats/min for the ten-year-old child to about
165 for the sixty-five-year-old adult. The reason for this decline
is unknown, but it certainly contributes to the decrease in maximal
VO_2 with age. There is another consequence of a lower maximal
heart rate. Studies on thirty-three building workers (bricklayers,
carpenters, laborers) from thirty to seventy years of age showed that
the mean heart rate during occupational activity was correlated with
the individual's maximal heart rate (Fig. 2-9). The person with
a high maximal heart rate of 185 beats/min can do a day's work

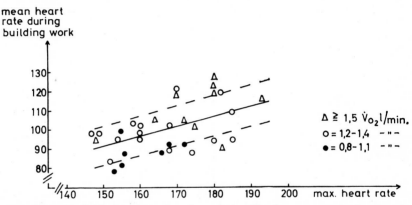

Figure 2-9. Individual values for the relationship between mean heart rate
during occupational work (building) and maximal heart rate attained during
work on bicycle ergometer. The heart rate was recorded by telemetry. The
estimated oxygen uptakes during occupational work are presented on the
right, together with their symbols. (From I. Åstrand, 1967, Courtesy of Taylor and Francis, Ltd.)

at a higher mean heart rate (110) than a person with a low maximal
heart rate of 150, who only reaches about 90 beats/min in the work
(I. Åstrand, 1967). However, the relative strain on the two persons
seems to be the same.

The maximal oxygen uptake does not only reveal the maximal
aerobic power of the individual, but it is also highly correlated to
his maximal cardiac output and stroke volume (Fig. 2-10).

DIMENSIONS

In a group of twenty-year to thirty-year-old well-trained women

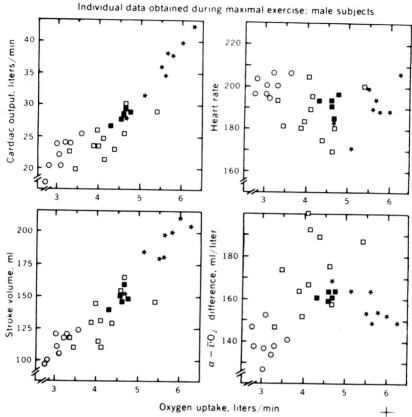

Individual data obtained during maximal exercise; male subjects

Figure 2-10. Cardiac output, heart rate, stroke volume, and arteriovenous oxygen difference during maximal exercise in relation to maximal oxygen uptake in top athletes who were very successful in endurance events (*stars*), well-trained but less successful athletes (*filled squares*), and twenty-five-year-old habitually sedentary subjects (*unfilled circles*). From Ekblom (1969). Included are maximal values on eleven well-trained physical education students (*unfilled squares*). (From Åstrand *et al.*, 1964.)

and men the maximal stroke volume was related to heart volume as expected from their dimensions (both being proportional to L^3 where L is body height); the maximal cardiac output was proportional to the heart volume raised to the 0.76 power, which is close to the expected 0.7 (for details see Åstrand and Rodahl, 1970). Maximal oxygen uptake is, however, lower than expected from the dimensions in women as well as children compared with adult men.

One explanation could be differences in hemoglobin concentration of the blood. In fact, young boys have only about 80 percent of the amount of hemoglobin of older boys per kilogram of body weight. However, the maximal oxygen uptake in children and young adults is proportional to the muscle strength and to Hb_T raised to the 0.76 power (Hb_T = total amount of hemoglobin), which is to be ex-

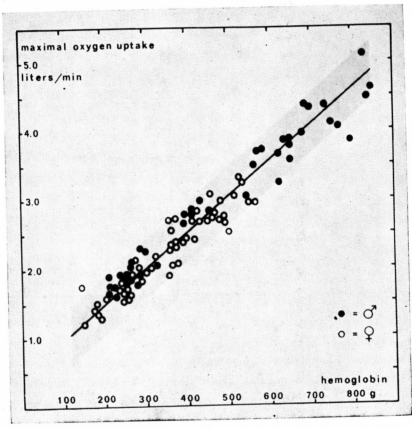

Figure 2-11. Maximal oxygen uptake for ninty-four subjects, age seven to thirty years, in relation to total amount of hemoglobin. In the equation $\dot{V}_{O_2}$ = a $\times$ $Hb_T{}^b$ the exponent b = 0.76. The subjects were all fairly well trained, and none of them was overweight. (For all subjects r = 0.979 $\pm$ 0.006; 2 $\times$ SD within shadowed area. For the determination of total hemoglobin, a CO method was used and the *absolute* values may be doubtful.) (From Åstrand and Rodahl, 1970, p. 332. Courtesy of McGraw-Hill Publishing Company.)

pected in geometrically similar and otherwise identical individuals of different sizes (Fig. 2-11).

Above the age of thirty there is, however, no longer a similar strict interrelation between statical and functional dimensions. In average, body height is maintained constant, but body weight, heart weight, and heart volume increase with age. Blood volume and total amount of hemoglobin are not markedly changed. Heart rate (and oxygen pulse) at a given submaximal work load is roughly the same in the old and the young. However, maximal oxygen uptake, heart rate, stroke volume, pulmonary ventilation, and muscular strength decrease significantly with age. Apparently an old individual of the same body size as a younger one is in many ways different both in structure and in function.

TRAINING

Because of limited space I will concentrate on one study and then present some principles for training. In Dallas, Chapman and co-workers conducted an extensive study on the effect of a twenty-day period of bed rest followed by a fifty-day period of physical training in five male subjects, aged nineteen to twenty-one (Saltin *et al.*, 1968). Three of the subjects had previously been sedentary, and two of them had been physically active, which may explain the difference in maximal oxygen uptake noticed in the control studies before the bed rest (Fig. 2-12). The maximal oxygen uptake fell from an average of 3.3 liters/min in the control study to 2.4 liters/min after bed rest, i.e. there was a 27 percent drop. After the training it was 3.9 liters/min or an average 18 percent higher than in the control study. Figure 2-13 summarizes the circulatory data. The stroke volume was much lower after the bed rest and highest in the trained subjects. Since there were no significant differences in maximal heart rate, the variation in stroke volume is reflected in marked modification of maximal cardiac output in the different states of training condition. An oxygen uptake that could normally be attained with a heart rate of 145 required a heart rate of 180 beats/min after bed rest. In this as well as in other studies on the effect of training (Ekblom, 1969) there is a dual basis for an increased maximal oxygen uptake: (a) an increased maximal cardiac output; (b) an in-

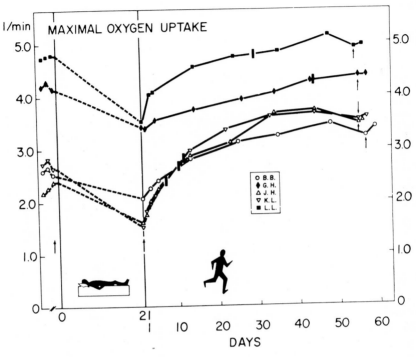

Figure 2-12. Changes in maximal oxygen uptake, measured during running on a treadmill, before and after bed rest and at various intervals during training; individual data on five subjects. Arrows indicate circulation studies. Heavy bars mark the time during the training period at which the maximal oxygen uptake had returned to the control value before bed rest. (From Saltin et al., 1968. Courtesy of American Heart Association.)

creased A-V O_2 difference. Quantitatively these two factors appear to contribute about equally towards increasing the maximal aerobic power. Figure 2-14 illustrates the dramatic improvement in maximal aerobic power noted in the three usually sedentary subjects, when comparing the "after bed rest" values with the posttraining ones. They actually increased their maximal oxygen uptake by 100 percent, or from 1.74 to an average of 3.41 liters/min.

This study by Saltin et al. illustrates how critical the level of physical activity before a training regime is for the evaluation of the effectiveness of a training program to improve the maximal $\dot{V}_{O_2}$. In the previously physically active subjects the improvement was

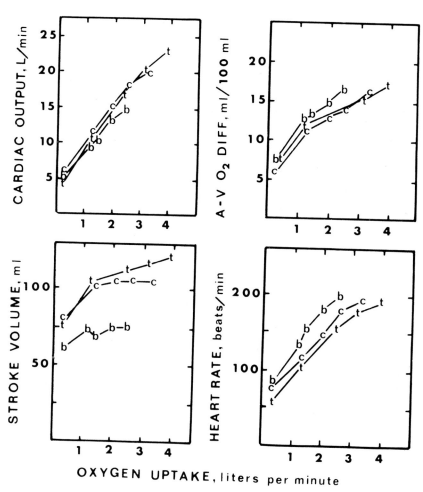

c = control; b = bed rest; t = training study; 5 subjects

Figure 2-13. Mean values of cardiac output, arteriovenous oxygen difference, stroke volume, and heart rate in relation to oxygen uptake during running at submaximal and maximal intensity before (c) and after (b) a twenty-day period of bed rest, and again after a fifty-day training (t). (Modified from Saltin *et al.*, 1968.)

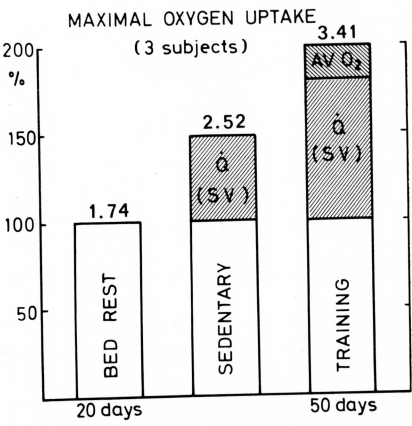

Figure 2-14. Maximal oxygen uptake during treadmill running for three subjects (1) after bed rest (= 100%), (2) when they are habitually sedentary, and (3) after intensive training, respectively. The higher oxygen uptake under sedentary conditions compared with bed rest is due to an increased maximal cardiac output (Q). The further increase after training is possible due to a further increase in maximal cardiac output and A-VO₂ difference. The maximal heart rate was the same throughout the experiment. Therefore, the increased cardiac output was due to a larger stroke volume (SV). (From Åstrand and Rodahl, 1970, p. 406, based on data from Saltin *et al.*, 1968. Courtesy of McGraw-Hill Book Publishing Company.)

only 4 percent. Starting with the "after bed rest" level, the increase was, however, 34 percent. In the three previously sedentary subjects the improvement was 33 and 100 percent, respectively. In other words, the training program applied may be said to have caused the maximal oxygen uptake of the participants to increase from 4 to 100 percent depending on how the initial level is defined.

Table 2-III summarizes data from various sources on variations in measured maximal oxygen uptake during prolonged bed rest and training, respectively, in longitudinal studies (training period up to 6 mos). Control values were obtained before bed rest and training. If not otherwise stated, subjects were twenty to thirty years of age.

With one exception the increase in maximal oxygen uptake with training was less than 20 percent. In the studies by Ekblom and

TABLE 2-III

Authors	*Number of Subjects*	*Maximal Oxygen Uptake, liters/minute*		
		Control	*After Bed Rest*	*After Training*
Robinson and Harmon				
1941 (Dill *et al.*, 1966)	9	3.36	. . . .	3.90 + 16%
Knehr *et al.*, 1942	14	3.45	. . . .	3.59 + 7%
Taylor *et al.*, 1949	2	3.85	3.18—17%	
Rowell, 1962	7	3.47	. . . .	3.93 + 13%
Ekblom *et al.*, 1968	8	3.15	. . . .	3.68 + 16%
Saltin *et al.*, 1968	3	2.52	1.74—31%	3.41 + 33%
Saltin *et al.*, 1969	42*	2.90	. . . .	3.43 + 18%
Saltin *et al.*, 1969	8†	2.25	. . . .	2.67 + 19%
I. Åstrand and Kilbom				
to be published	11‡	1.90	. . . .	2.18 + 15%

* Age thirty-four to fifty years.
† Age fifty to sixty-three years.
‡ Women, age nineteen to twenty-seven years.
(For complete reference list see Åstrand and Rodahl, 1970, Chapter 12.)

Saltin and co-workers the training often included maximal efforts. I. Åstrand and Kilbom let their subjects train three half-hours weekly with three-minute work periods, interrupted by resting periods of two minutes. All training was performed on bicycle ergometers, and the work was definitely submaximal (heart rate up to resting level + 70 percent of difference between resting level and maximal heart rate). The improvement was as high as 15 percent.

PRINCIPLES FOR TRAINING

An adaptation to a given load takes place gradually; in order to achieve further improvement the training intensity has to be increased. (a) There is, however, no linear relationship between amount of training and the training effect. For instance, two hours of training per week may cause an increase in maximal O_2 uptake, by 0.4 liter/min. If the training is twice as much, that is, four hours per week, the increase in O_2 uptake will not be twice as great, that is 0.8 liter/min, but possibly 0.5 to 0.6 liter/min. Obviously there is a limit to the increase, and the rate and magnitude of the increase varies from one individual to the next. It is important to ascertain, in one way or the other, what amount of training may produce a satisfactory result. (b) Older individuals may be less trainable than younger ones. On the other hand, some effect of training can be noticed even at very old age. (c) Less effort is demanded to maintain a reasonable degree of physical condition than to attain it after a period of prolonged activity.

Physical activity ranging from repeated work periods of a few seconds duration up to hours of continuous work may involve a major load on the oxygen-transporting organs and thereby induce a training effect. The following method appears to be more "foolproof" than most other methods. One should work with large muscle groups for three to five minutes, rest or engage in light physical activity for some minutes, then proceed with a further work period, etc., as required, depending on ambitions and the objective of the training. For most of us two to three half-hours weekly will probably be rather optimal. Actually, the tempo shall not be maximal during the work periods. When the oxygen uptake reaches maximal levels the cardiac output and stroke volume are also maximum. A further increase in work intensity is possible thanks to an anaerobic energy yield, but the cardiac output and stroke volume may even be somewhat reduced. Certainly the work becomes very exhausting and straining. In other words, since maximal oxygen uptake and cardiac output can be attained at a submaximal speed, this lower speed is probably optimal as a training stimulus. As pointed out, even work loads demanding only a submaximal oxygen uptake do improve the physical condition for very untrained individuals. Anyone who wants to increase his anaerobic power must on the other hand perform all-out efforts, but this is in my opinion of small interest for nonathletes.

Because of limited time I can only summarize the main components of a rational training program aimed at developing the different types of power:

(1) Bursts of intense activity lasting only a few seconds may develop muscle strength and stronger tendons and ligaments.

(2) Intense activity lasting for about one minute, repeated after about four minutes of rest or mild exercise, etc. may develop the anaerobic power.

(3) Activity with large muscles involved, less than maximal intensity, for about three to five minutes, repeated after rest or mild exercise of similar duration may develop the aerobic power.

(4) Activity at submaximal intensity lasting as long as thirty minutes or more may develop endurance, i.e. the ability to tax a larger percentage of the individual's maximal aerobic power.

(For details see Åstrand and Rodahl, 1970, Chapter 12.)

TESTS OF PHYSICAL CONDITION

Objective tests to determine the effect of training on different functions are both important and desirable. Such tests may be an aid in the development of the program, and they encourage the individual to continue his training. In my opinion the submaximal bicycle ergometer test is the simplest, cheapest, and most reliable one. In longitudinal studies it is an advantage to apply a test where variations in body weight do not complicate the choice of work load, and in this connection the bicycle ergometer is superior to treadmill or step tests. For children below the age of about ten the treadmill must, however, be the preferred tool. With exception for very specific research projects, it is unrealistic and unwise to include maximal physical efforts in testing procedures. I also want to point out that that most of the so-called fitness tests, including evaluation of flexibility, skill, strength, etc. are usually related to special gymnastic or athletic performance; they are really not suitable for an analysis of basic physiological functions. The widespread use of such test batteries in physical education can be justified from a pedagogic and psychological viewpoint. However, from medical and physio-

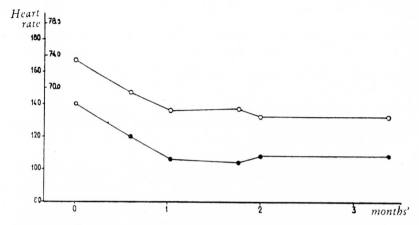

Figure 2-15. Decrease in heart rate tested at two fixed work loads in the course of three and one-half months of training. Work intensity 600 kpm (*filled circles*) and 900 kpm (*open circles*).

logical aspects, application of a test battery or, for instance, a trial of the distance that can be covered within twelve minutes may be unsuitable, since the performance of the tests usually demands maximal exertion of a subject who may be completely untrained.

Figure 2-15 illustrates the application of a submaximal work test during a period of training. The same test can be applied in top athletes, in trained and untrained adults, and in children older than about ten years of age. The individual is his own control; it is a matter of comparing the individual with himself at repeated tests over months or years. It should be emphasized again that the individual's maximal oxygen uptake, heart size, or heart rate at a single submaximal test does not reveal anything about his state of training, since constitutional factors play a greater role than merely the state of training. A person may have a low heart rate at a standard load and yet be entirely untrained, and a well-trained individual may show a high heart rate.

It has been recently observed by Hartley and Saltin (1968) that untrained subjects who (a) work for six minutes at an O_2 uptake of about 40 percent of their maximal aerobic power, then (b) work for six minutes at a load of about 70 percent of their maximum, followed by (c) a ten-minute rest, and then (d) repeat the 40 percent load, now have the same O_2 uptake and cardiac output as under (a), but they have now a significantly higher heart rate, in many cases as much as 20 beats/min higher. Following training, this increase in heart rate becomes less, and well-trained athletes may accomplish the entire procedure listed above with the results from (a) and (d) being almost identical. This type of testing appears quite promising as a method of objectively assessing the level of physical condition and habitual physical exercise.

PREDICTION OF MAXIMAL OXYGEN UPTAKE

Most exercise tests for an evaluation of physical work capacity or, more specific, maximal oxygen uptake, are based on a linear increase in heart rate with increasing O_2 uptake or work load. However, all predictions from submaximal tests should be done with the utmost caution. When persons of different age groups are included, some sort of correction factor must be included since the maximal heart rate declines with age (*cf*. I. Åstrand, 1960). Even when the tests are carried out during strictly standardized conditions, the methodological error in a prediction of the maximal aerobic power is considerable (SD $= 10\%$ to 15%). They can, however, be applied as a valuable screening test for the evaluation of the functional capacity of the oxygen-transporting system; they may provide a useful method for selecting out the best, the worst, and the average men from a group.

WORK TESTS ON PATIENTS

In the examination of patients an exercise test makes it possible to include observations and studies during physical activity which may simulate the work load at the patient's daily activities. Figure 2-16 provides a help in the choice of suitable work load on a bicycle ergometer. Heart size, ECG, blood pressure, etc. should be evaluated together with results from the work test. In the Scandinavian countries one has agreed about this general procedure: The subject (or patient) is exposed to work loads on the bicycle ergometer for six-minute periods, starting with a low load and increasing the load in a stepwise fashion. The aim is to increase the load until the subject's heart rate has reached a certain level related to the maximal heart

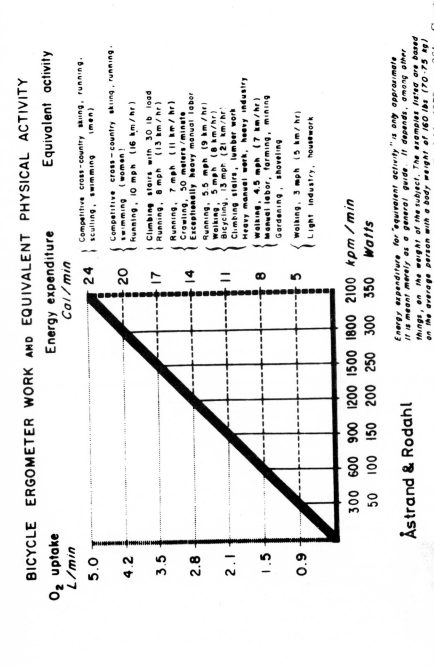

Figure 2-16. Bicycle ergometer work and equivalent physical activity. (From Åstrand and Rodahl, 1970, p. 364. Courtesy of McGraw-Hill Book Publishing Company.)

rate that is typical for his age (actual mean value – 2.5 SD). With a limit for young persons twenty to twenty-nine years of age at a heart rate of 170 beats/min it should be 160 per minute for thirty to thity-nine years old, 150 per minute for forty to forty-nine years old, 140 per minute for fifty to fifty-nine years old, and 130 per minute for sixty to sixty-nine years old (I. Åstrand *et al.*, 1967). A test performed in this fashion permits, for instance, a classification of the ECG both at a fixed load independent of the individual's work capacity, and at a load related to the individual's circulatory capacity. Other advantages with this procedure are that (a) the test is easy to perform, and (b) the physical demands of different occupational or recreational activities can be reproduced.

It is very difficult to summarize a paper which has tried to summarize about a dozen different aspects of aerobic power. I just conclude by emphasizing that physical conditioning can effectively improve the aerobic power, and fortunately it is not necessary to work hard to obtain good results. It is fortunate because most of us, including me, do not like it when it hurts.

REFERENCES

1. Åstrand, I.: Aerobic work capacity in men and women with special reference to age. *Acta Physiol Scand,* Vol. 49, Suppl. 169, 1960.
2. Åstrand I.: Degree of strain during building work as related to individual aerobic work capacity. *Ergonomics, 10:*293, 1967.
3. Åstrand, I. *et al.*: The "Minnesota Code" for ECG classification. Adaptation to CR leads and modification of the code for ECG's recorded during and after exercise. *Acta Med Scand,* Suppl. 481, 1967.
4. Åstrand, P.-O., and Christensen, E. H.: Aerobic work capacity. In F. Dickens, Neil, E., and Widdas, W. F. (Eds.): *Oxygen in the Animal Organism.* New York, Pergamon Press, 1964, P. 295.
5. Åstrand, P.-O., Cuddy, T. E., Saltin, B., and Stenberg, J.: Cardiac output during submaximal and maximal work. *J Appl Physiol, 19:* 268, 1964.
6. Åstrand, P.-O., and Rodahl, K.: *Textbook of Work Physiology.* New York, McGraw-Hill, 1970.
7. Bergström, J., and Hultman, E.: Muscle glycogen synthesis after exercise: An enhancing factor localized to the muscle cells in Man. *Nature, 210:*309, 1966.
8. Ekblom, B.: Effect of physical training on oxygen transport system in Man. *Acta Physiol Scand,* Suppl. 328, 1969.
9. Hansson, J.-E.: The relationship between individual characteristics of

the worker and output of work in logging operations. *Studia Forestalia Suecia,* no. 29, Skogshögskolan, Stockholm, 1965.

10. Hartley, L. H., and Saltin, B.: Reduction of stroke volume and increase in heart rate after a previous heavier submaximal work load. *Scand J Clin Lab Invest, 22*:217, 1968.

11. Hermansen, L., and Saltin, B.: Oxygen uptake during maximal treadmill and bicycle exercise. *J Appl Physiol. 26*:31, 1969.

12. Saltin, B., Blomqvist, G., Mitchell, J. H., Johnson Jr., R. L., Wildenthal, K., and Chapman, C. B.: Response to submaximal and maximal exercise after bed rest and training. *Circulation,* Vol. 38, Suppl. 7, 1968.

Chapter 3

PROGRAMS OF EXERCISE–
PHYSIOLOGICAL CONSIDERATIONS

HOWARD G. KNUTTGEN

Whenever the terms "fitness" or "fitness program" are used, the specific objectives which are desired must be described. In other words, the question must be answered, "fitness for what?" There are many anatomical, physiological, and psychological factors which determine a person's fitness for various types of physical activity, and in turn, each physical activity requires different combinations of these features. I emphasize this because, in response to a physician's general admonition to "get some exercise," a person might think of taking up weight lifting, tennis, or jogging. Each activity would place a different set of stresses on the body, as each activity requires a different set of capacities. Continuous participation in any of the three would bring about different physiological changes in the person, and therefore, quite different types of fitness.

Considering all the possibilities of physical performance, the various factors which determine a person's capacity for different activities could be arranged in the following categories (for a full discussion of these catgories, see reference 15):

1. Physical size and body proportions
2. Energy release processes
3. Energy sources available
4. Strengths
5. Speeds of movement
6. Skills
7. Psychological factors

Certain of these categories bear little relationship to fitness for the various activities of daily living and the maintenance of general health for the adult male group we are considering in this symposium. I would suggest, therefore, that the objectives of an adult activity

[53]

program, which gives especial attention to the maintenance or improvement of the functional capacity of the circulatory system, could most probably be divided into three headings: coordination and skills, body weight control, and aerobic capacity.

COORDINATION AND SKILLS

Providing an individual has the strengths adequate to a task (e.g. moving around a handball court or shooting a basketball), it remains only for him to teach his nervous system how to control and coordinate the various muscular contractions in order to perform the task successfully. If the participants in the type of program under consideration do not have skills necessary for the activities planned, it would certainly be worthwhile to include and combine skill teaching into the routine of each session. As participation in competitive sports, such as handball, squash racquets, paddle ball, tennis, and the like, would aid in the attainment of the other objectives we will consider, this would be further reason to include skills instruction in the overall program. Coordination and skills as an objective should not necessarily be considered as an end but rather as a means to another end, namely the ability to participate in physical activity.

BODY WEIGHT CONTROL

The contribution of exercise to body weight control has frequently been questioned and even discredited. Such reasoning can apparently be justified if one attempts to calculate the possible weight loss (other than by sweating) in a single bout of exercise. It is, as a matter of fact, surprisingly small. A sizeable weight loss can be found, however, if one calculates the total amount of fuel necessary to sustain moderate to heavy exercise sessions for one hour every other day for a year. It is further evident that it is the proper combination of daily food intake and daily energy release which dominates the control of body weight.

AEROBIC CAPACITY

The focus of this symposium is on the relationship of exercise to the heart, and therefore, emphasis must be given to what is usually referred to as aerobic activity. We can define aerobic muscular activity as any activity which is made possible by a constant supply of oxygen being delivered from the lungs to active muscle cells. This type of activity is not characterized by short bursts but rather by extended duration, anywhere from two minutes to more than an hour, if desired.

As was emphasized by both Dr. Rowell and Dr. Åstrand, capacity for endurance-type activity is dependent upon the capacity for continuous oxygen delivery, and oxygen delivery is, in turn, dependent upon circulatory factors. If the functional capacity of the circulatory system either deteriorates or improves, the functional capacity of the individual changes accordingly with respect to performance of endurance-type activity. If this functional capacity of the circulatory system is maintained at a high level, the individual is assured of a greater capacity for daily activity and, also, that the stresses of submaximal physical work and sport will constitute relatively lower levels of stress. The role of exercise in cardiovascular disease prevention is less clear, but indications are strong that the relationship is both positive and significant.

In order to improve functional capacity of the circulatory system and improve aerobic capacity, one must stress the oxygen transport system with periods of exercise which demand relatively large amounts of oxygen. Little or no benefit in this regard results from activities which do not tax the oxygen transport system, such as walking, golf, weight lifting, isometrics, or competitive sports where activity takes place in short spurts. Improvement in aerobic capacity results from repeated participation at relatively intense levels in activities such as jogging, running, swimming, cycling, continuous calisthenics, or competitive sports where gross activity is maintained at a high level for extended periods.

If the activities mentioned are carried on for extended periods and at moderate to heavy levels of stress, this means a considerable release of energy and, therefore, the consumption of considerable quantities of energy stores in the body. Therefore, participation in endurance type or aerobic activities can go hand in hand with body weight control.

The results of various exercise regimens for development of aerobic capacity and/or control of body weight which have been examined by controlled investigation bear some differences because of variations in the activities or program protocols employed (1, 2, 5a, 5b, 6-10, 14, 16-19, 21). If we pool all of the results and conclusions, certain general recommendations regarding exercise programs emerge:

1. Participation should occur two to three times per week as a minimum, with greater improvement expected as a result of more frequent participation.
2. Activities should be "oxygen-demanding" in nature and carried on at an intensity level which could be described as moderate to heavy (e.g. heart rates sustained for periods of 5 to 15 min at 120 to 160 beats/min).
3. Each exercise period should last from thirty to sixty minutes.
4. Bouts of oxygen-demanding activity might very well be interspersed with periods of skill instruction.
5. The level of intensity and the length of the exercise period for any single participant should be determined by his health history, his level of condition (e.g. as evaluated by cycle ergometer or step test), and his personal objectives.

These considerations relate only to exercise. I would like to suggest, however, that a fitness program should include more than participation in physical activity. The participants should be aided in understanding the contribution of exercise to a total concept of health and well-being, which would include improved functional capacity as one factor in general health. The fitness program could very well include the dissemination of information concerning the interrelationships of general health, exercise, diet, rest, and relaxation. A person who participates in an exercise program and still overeats, does not obtain appropriate nutriments, does not get sufficient rest, or leads a tension-filled existence may well be wasting his time as far as attainment of a better state of health is concerned. Therefore, the fitness program leader should be well informed as to the full meaning of the concept of health and should conduct his program with this full meaning firmly in mind.

ENVIRONMENTAL CONDITIONS

In planning and conducting an exercise program, one must consider more than the aerobic capacity of the participants and the types and levels of activity appropriate to the objectives. It is quite possible to add to the stress that the metabolic demand of exercise places on the body by adding a thermal stress. During physical exercise, most of the calories of energy released in the muscle cells are not related to the energetics of body movement but are given off from the cells as heat. This heat must be dissipated from the body in order to maintain the body temperature within a tolerable limit for the nervous system and so as not to impose an undue thermal load on the circulatory system.

The exercising man can lose heat by means of evaporation of sweat from the skin, by radiation (giving off infrared rays), and by conduction-convection (passing heat to air moving past the body). It is, however, the evaporative mechanism that bears most of the responsibility during vigorous exercise. In order for the sweating process to be effective, the sweat must evaporate. Beads of sweat dripping from a person are less effective in heat dissipation, and their appearance constitutes an important warning sign of the possible inability of the body to lose heat rapidly because of ambient conditions. In order for all three mechanisms to be effective, the skin surface must be sufficiently exposed.

An exercising man can even gain heat if the air temperature is higher than his body temperature (which is a distinct possibility in the United States during the summer months) or if he is exposed to infrared radiation. The latter could come from the sun or from heated objects, such as walls or pavements exposed to the sun.

Participants should not wear excessive clothing when exercising, especially when the environment is comfortable. Shorts and T-shirts should be all that is necessary. Sweatsuits and other such apparel severely inhibit the various heat loss processes and should only be used in cool or cold environments. Whenever necessary, comfortable air circulation should be induced in indoor facilities so as to aid the movement of air around the participants and to maintain a pleasant environment.

As a sidelight, there is no evidence to indicate that elevating the body temperature "burns off" body fat. The weight loss resulting from excessive sweating because of the wearing of excessive clothing (sweatsuits and oilskins) is merely a water loss and does not affect the body fat content. This weight can be immediately regained by drinking a glass of water.

The evaluation of an environment as to its suitability for strenuous activity is best accomplished by measurement of the air temperature, humidity, infrared radiation, and air movement. Such measurements and the calculation of such factors as the partial pressure of water vapor in the air are somewhat intricate, and most attempts at simple indices for curtailing physical activity have not been successful. The exercise leader should keep in mind the danger of the double stress of exercise and thermal load and curtail activity when either the air temperature is high or, especially, if both the air temperature and relative humidity are high. A good index of the suitability of the environment in these respects is the general appearance of the participants and their own subjective evaluation of the comfort of the environment.

None of the physiologic parameters, such as heart rate, cardiac output, sweat rate, or body temperature, shows direct relationship to external heat load or internal heat production if (a) either of these two factors are allowed to vary independently or (b) other factors are not held constant. If certain levels of activity are accepted as typical for an exercise session, one can make a prediction of the temperature and humidity conditions that could make the environment uncomfortable and, possibly, a threat to the well-being of the participants.

Dr. Karel Lustinec, of the Institute of Industrial Hygiene and Occupational Diseases (Prague), has kindly provided two charts for such prediction (12), one for exercise sessions which would be described as light to moderate in intensity and the other for sessions described as moderate to heavy in intensity. (See Figs. 3-1 and 3-2.) Measurement must be made of both the dry bulb air temperature and the wet bulb air temperature (the latter performed so as to include the effect of ambient water vapor tension). This can be performed very rapidly and easily with an inexpensive apparatus, the sling psychrometer, which is available from any general scientific supply house. When the two temperatures have been determined, the exercise leader may refer to the appropriate chart to determine

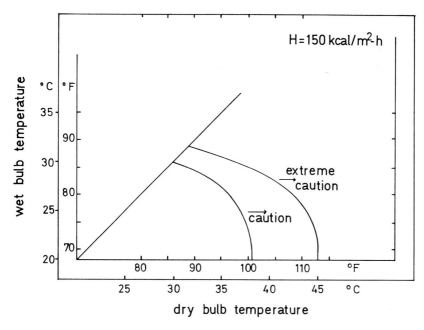

Figure 3-1. Chart for determining environmental conditions under which caution should be taken when the level of exercise is light to moderate (heat production of 150 kcal per square meter body surface area per hour). Line of identity represents 100 percent relative humidity. (Chart constructed from data in references 11 and 13.)

if their intersect lies to the right of the lines labeled "Caution" or "Extreme Caution." These charts are presented not as absolute standards that would dictate alteration or cancellation of an exercise session, but rather as an aid to the conscientious exercise leader.

TESTING

The testing of skills will not be discussed at any length. It should be sufficient to mention that, if skill improvement is an objective, skill testing by standard or self-devised tests of the program director could certainly add interest to the total program. Frequent recording of body weight is a simple and worthwhile inclusion in the routine of the program, perhaps on a weekly basis.

Direct measurement of a person's aerobic capacity (maximum ability to take up and utilize oxygen) involves expense and laboratory

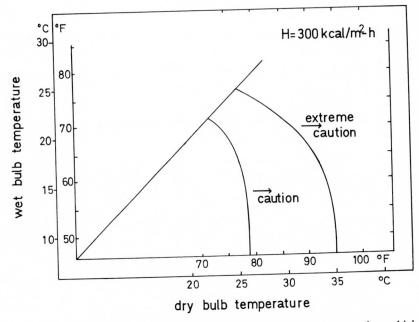

Figure 3-2. Chart for determining environmental conditions under which caution should be taken when the level of exercise is moderate to heavy (heat production of 300 kcal per square meter body surface area per hour). (Chart constructed from data in references 11 and 13.)

technology, discomfort to the person being tested, and possible dangers to any cardiac risk participants. Indirect measurement, as described by Dr. Åstrand, involves some basic knowledge of the physiological factors involved, a modest amount of equipment, care in testing protocol, and consideration of the limitations of indirect methods (3, 4, 20). At the very least, such indirect measurements (or prediction) can give an indication of the person's physiological fitness for endurance-type work and periodic retesting can give indication of improvement. Such evaluation also constitutes a strong motivational tool for the participants.

Any time objectives are set forth for an exercise program, it should be possible for the program director to measure progress being made toward attaining these objectives. Periodic notation of body weight measured with an accurate balance can quickly determine success in maintaining or attaining suitable body weight. Determination of steady-state heart rate during bicycle ergometer exercise or recovery heart rate from a step test can certainly furnish an adequate index of initial level of physical condition and of progress toward the objective of increased circulatory function and aerobic capacity.

In my opinion, no exercise program director should include the term "fitness" to name or describe his program unless he has the equipment, ability, and intention of evaluating the reaction of the circulatory system to controlled exercise.

REFERENCES

1. Buskirk, E. R., Thompson, R., Lutwak, L., and Whedon, G.: Energy balance of obese patients during weight reduction: Influence of diet and exercise. *Ann NY Acad Sci, 110*:918-940, 1963.

2. Cureton, T., and Phillips, E.: Physical fitness changes in middle-aged men attributable to equal eight-week periods of training, non-training, and retraining. *J Sports Med, 4*:87-93, 1964.

3. Davies, C. T. M.: Limitations to the prediction of maximum oxygen uptake from cardiac frequency measurements. *J Appl Physiol, 24*:700-706, 1968.

4. de Vries, H. A., and Klafs, C. E.: Prediction of oxygen uptake from submaximal tests. *J Sports Med, 5*:207-214, 1965.

5a Ekblom, B.: Effect of physical training on oxygen transport in man. *Acta Physiol Scand,* Suppl. 328, 1969.

5b Ekblom, B.: Effect of physical training in adolescent boys. *J Appl Physiol, 27*:350-355, 1969.

6. Ekblom, B., Åstrand, P.-O., Saltin, B., Stenberg, J., and Wallstrom, B.: Effect of training on circulatory response to exercise. *J Appl Physiol, 24*:518-528, 1968.

7. Grimby, G., and Saltin, B.: Physiological analyses of physically well-trained middle-aged and old athletes. *Acta Med Scand, 179:513-526,* 1966.

8. Hartley, L. H., Åstrand, I., Kihlbom, A., Ekblom, B., and Saltin, B.: Improvement of maximal oxygen uptake and cardiac output by physical training in sedentary middle-aged men. *In Proceedings of the International Union of Physiological Sciences.* Washington, D. C., XXIV International Congress, 1968, Vol. VII, p. 183.

9. Hanson, J. S., Tabakin, B. S., Levy, A. M., and Nedde, W.: Long-term physical training and cardiovascular dynamics in middle aged men. *Circulation, 38*:783-799, 1968.

10. Holmgren, A., Mossfeldt, F., Sjostrand, T., and Strom, G.: Effect of training on work capacity, total hemoglobin, blood volume, heart

volume, and pulse rate in recumbent and upright position. *Acta Physiol Scand, 50:*72-83, 1960.

11. Lustinec, K.: The working microclimate and its evalution. *Informational News from Industrial Hygiene (Institute of Industrial Hygiene and Occupational Diseases),* Vol. 13, Suppl. 2, 1967.

12. Lustinec, K.: (Institute of Industrial Hygiene and Occupational Diseases, Prague). Personal Communication.

13. Lofstedt, B.: *Human Heat Tolerance.* Lund: Berlingska Boktryckeriet, 1966.

14. Karlsson, J., Åstrand, P.-O., Ekblom, B.: Training of the oxygen transport system in man. *J Appl Physiol, 22:*1061-1065, 1967.

15. Knuttgen, H. G.: Physical working capacity and physical performance (Symposium on the Physiological Basis for Human Work Performance). *Med Sci Sports, 1:*1-8, 1969.

16. Moody, D. L., Kollias, J., and Buskirk, E. R.: The effect of a moderate exercise program on body weight and skinfold thickness in overweight college women. *Med Sci Sports, 1:*75-80, 1969.

17. Naughton, J., and Balke, B.: Physical working capacity in medical personnel and the response of serum cholesterol to acute exercise and training. *Amer J Med Sci, 247:*286-292, 1964.

18. Naughton, J., and Nagle, F.: Peak oxygen intake during physical fitness program for middle-aged men. *JAMA, 191:*899-901, 1965.

19. Pollock, M. L., Cureton, T. K., and Greninger, L.: Effects of training on working capacity, cardiovascular function, and body composition of adult men. *Med Sci Sports, 1:*70-74, 1969.

20. Rowell, L. B., Taylor, H. L., and Wang, Y.: Limitations to prediction of maximal oxygen intake. *J Appl Physiol, 19:*919-927, 1964.

21. Saltin, B., Blomquist, B., Mitchell, J. H., Johnsson, R., Wildenthal, K., and Chapman, C. B.: Response to submaximal and maximal exercise after bed rest and training. *Circulation,* Vol. 38, Suppl. 7, 1968.

Chapter 4

PROGRAMS OF EXERCISE—
PROGRAM ORGANIZATION

LAWRENCE A. GOLDING

Iₙ ᴀ ᴄᴏɴꜰᴇʀᴇɴᴄᴇ such as this, it may at first seem somewhat un-
sophisticated to talk about the actual exercises that one must do in
order to accomplish the results that are being presented here today.
Yet, in one sense, the program is the most important part of physical
conditioning, because it is the program that is followed—the actual
exercises that are done—that enable us to enjoy the beneficial effects
that come from activity. Without a successful program, without a
successful means of getting people to exercise regularly, optimum
results cannot be achieved.

I would like then, to talk about some of the considerations involved in organizing a program of exercise.

From my own experience, I know that the average group of
middle-aged adults who are interested in physical fitness are athletically
unskilled. They are not ex-athletes who want to get back into shape;
they are not individuals who are particularly interested in playing
games or learning and developing athletic skills. They are, primarily,
sedentary individuals who have heard about, and been impressed by,
the fact that inactivity is harmful, that sedentary living is a coronary
risk factor, that it results in degenerative diseases, that it decreases
one's physical working capacity, and that it makes one physiologically
old at a chronologically youthful age. This individual may not like,
nor really want to exercise, but he is sometimes frightened by the
high incidence of coronary artery disease in relatively young men
and is, therefore, highly motivated. Calisthenics, bicycling, jogging,
etc. are not only appealing but valuable and practical for our fitness enthusiasts because these activities do not involve any high level
of skill, or any expensive equipment. On the other hand, volleyball,

[63]

basketball, handball, tennis, etc. may be more fun, and when played competitively may be fitness producing, but one must have a high level of skill to attain the necessary values from these activities. So the general physical fitness class that we see in the YMCA is designed for and well-suited to the vast majority of middle-aged adults.

Although many health clubs can provide everything necessary for the individual who wishes to get into better physical condition, these clubs are seldom successful because, while the individual is told what to do, given facilities and equipment, the clubs provide little or no leadership. We know that exercise is not particularly easy and many times not even enjoyable, and it becomes almost impossible psychologically to do alone. A few individuals may have enough motivation and self-discipline to exercise alone, but most of us last only a few days or, at the most, a few weeks, after which a dozen conflicts cause us to gradually become more and more irregular, until we finally stop altogether.

A class, with trained leadership offers an external discipline, a social pressure, and a stated committment that keeps individuals exercising. So the typical YMCA physical fitness class which meets regularly, checks attendance, and has trained leadership, is probably the best form an exercise program can take.

A good exercise program has three basic components. The first is the warm-up period. This is when the muscles are stretched and joints put through their full range of motion. This period of preparation involves bending, stretching, and twisting exercises. After the warm-up the skeletal muscles are exercised—both for strength and endurance. This second part of a well rounded exercise program, then, consists of activities such as sit-ups, push-ups, chins, etc. Although calisthenics are sometimes frowned upon by professional physical educators, seven or eight well chosen calisthenics will efficiently and systematically exercise each major muscle group of the body.

Before going to the third part of an exercise program, let me say something about calisthenics and strength development. Today, most of the emphasis of researchers and physical educators is on cardiovascular fitness—increasing the efficiency of the heart, circulation, and lungs. We realize that skeletal muscle development is not a major factor in the prevention of degenerative disease. However, a few points need to be made in favor of calisthenics. Again, it must be remembered that calisthenics are only a part of the total program and are not designed to replace any type of endurance activity. Nevertheless, calisthenics can be beneficial from a number of standpoints: (a) A well-balanced physical fitness program should produce muscular fitness as well as cardiovascular fitness. (b) Esthetically, and functionally, it is desirable to have a flat abdomen and toned, well-developed muscles, and the cardiovascular type activity is not designed for this purpose. (c) One should have enough strength to take care of emergency situations. Although we are surrounded by labor saving devices, we still occasionally have to exert our muscles. (d) Running necessitates the development of the legs, but does not take care of the arms, shoulders, back, and abdomen. Runners often complain about low back pain, which might well be eliminated with well-designed back exercises to strengthen and condition these important muscles. (e) Calisthenics done repetitively without rest for fifteen minutes can quickly become a cardiovascular activity, therefore adding to our main interest of cardiovascular efficiency.

Physical directors often complain that once men start jogging, they no longer want to do calisthenics or, for that matter, any other form of exercise. As physical educators, we should stress a well-rounded, balanced program of exercise.

To continue with the components of a good exercise program, after a warm-up and a period devoted to muscular development, the third and most important part of an exercise program is the cardiovascular conditioning. Probably, the two best cardiovascular exercises are running and swimming.

Because I have suggested these three components of a good exercise program, I do not imply that they must be done in order. Obviously, the warm-up period must be first, but calisthenics can be mixed with running. In our program at Kent State University, we exercise on the football field where we do our calisthenics under the goal posts and then run the length of the field between each calisthenic. Any number of exercise routines can be developed with a little ingenuity. Weight lifting is a good activity for strength development, but it is too difficult to implement in a large class. Weight lifting is, more or less, an individual activity. Calisthenics, using the body weight as resistance, can be used more efficiently in a large group.

I know that many of you here today are involved in running programs, and what I am going to say will be echoed by most of you. In the final analysis, the exercise program is only as good as its leader. The YMCA should be congratulated on the excellent leadership it provides. Part of my job is to train physical educators for the public school systems, and I am dismayed at the quality of physcial fitness leadership in the physical education programs on the public school level—as evidenced by the number of physical educators who are, themselves, unfit. You cannot sell fitness with any success if you follow the "don't do as I do, do as I say" method of teaching. I see very few YMCA physical directors who are not involved in their own exercise programs and who are not fit. If you are sold on fitness, your enthusiasm and interest will be contagious and will spread to your classes or the individuals with whom you talk. You must believe in fitness enough to do something about it yourself.

Physical change comes from hard work progressively and persistently done. There are no secret exercises, no secret ingredients. No fads, gimmicks, or cults can replace perseverance and hard work. The attainment of physical fitness is relatively simple—namely gradually presenting the body with more and more work, progressing slowly but steadily, until some desirable level of fitness is attained, and then, being satisfied with that level, maintaining it with a regular program of work. We are not in the business of developing Olympic athletes. Our progressive work does not end only in the four-minute mile, but rather in helping individuals attain a level of fitness that can be measured and determined as adequate.

The physician who finds himself faced with the problem of prescribing exercises might well look for help to the physical educator, for he, like the physician, is becoming more knowledgeable in regard to the physiological effects of exercise. The local YMCA, if it has a good physical fitness program which includes testing and medical supervision, may well be the easiest answer for the physician. He can suggest that his patient enroll in the YMCA program. If the patient has no pathological problems and his physician feels that some regular exercise may be good preventive medicine, a well-designed exercise program may well be all he needs to recommend. In some communities the YMCA offers a postcoronary exercise program. If this is properly supervised it is invaluable for the physicians' postcoronary patients. But what about when there is no YMCA or any other organized program? Then he must prescribe the exercise himself. Some programs are available, such as the aerobics program, or the 5BX, or the program suggested by the President's Council on Adult Fitness, or a dozen other available books.

It is not within the realm of this presentation to outline exercises that may be used in an exercise program. And may I reemphasize that there is not one "best" exercise, no secret exercise, that will give the best results. Many times people have written asking for the list of exercises we use in our program, as though the ones we use are special or scientific. The secret is doing the exercises regularly and including a warm-up, some calisthenics and some cardiovascular activity, and having a good leader.

Getting people to do the exercises daily is the difficult part—and without a group or class it becomes even more difficult.

Recently much emphasis has been placed on marathon running. Hundred-mile clubs and thousand-mile clubs are good motivational devices. However, the concept that running ten, twenty, or thirty miles a day is necessary for fitness is unsound. One does not have to run ten or more miles a day to be fit. Overload can be imposed by intensity as well as duration. It becomes a serious question as to whether the ten-mile and twenty-mile run is not more an orthopedic stress than a cardiovascular one. Cults too often overlook the basic concepts of fitness. Good leadership implies a safe, well-supervised, carefully prescribed program.

Much of the leadership and guidelines for the local Y's should be coming from the National YMCA, but at present leadership in physical fitness and programming on the national level is sadly lacking. Therefore, today, excellent fitness programs in the Y are more dependent upon local physical directors than upon national leadership.

It is not my assignment to discuss testing, other than as it applies to class organization. What I say, therefore, will be cursory and brief. Testing in an exercise program is important because it does three things:

(1) It shows the subject how he compares to the general population.

(2) It motivates him to work so that measurable changes can result.

(3) It shows him the change that results from the exercise program.

A real distinction should be made between the kind of testing done in most YMCA's (which is program-oriented) and the testing which occurs in universities or hospitals where research is being conducted. Testing as performed in the Y is for the subject's own edification and is used to motivate the subject. Reliability, validity, or even accuracy, although highly desirable, are not the major concerns. In research, however, reliability, validity, and accuracy are the most important factors. I question whether ECG's, hydrostatic weighing or energy metabolism techniques belong in the YMCA; but, certainly, anthropometrical measurements; strength measurements; agility, balance, and flexibility measurements; vital capacity, and the PWC170 are highly beneficial for the general exercise program found in the YMCA. The bulk of the time should be spent on the program and not on the testing. Testing is only a tool to enhance the program.

In summary, I would like to repeat the major parts of this presentation.

1. A class situation with a trained, motivated, respected, and enthusiastic leader is one of the best ways in keeping the class successful.

2. A good program of exercise involves a warm-up or preparatory period of loosening-up exercises. And certainly, the older the group, the longer this period should be.

3. Calisthenics aimed at the skeletal muscles for both strength and muscular endurance should not be forgotten or eliminated. Although cardiovascular activities are of prime importance, skeletal muscle improvement should be included in a good program.

4. Running and swimming are two of the best cardiovascular

activities and should be done regularly and progressively. Increasing the intensity of the exercise can result in a high level of fitness.

5. Testing enables an individual to see how he is progressing and may even determine the level an individual may reach when he will be satisfied with his fitness level and work simply to maintain it.

6. Preferably, exercise should be preventive, and much of the emphasis of the professional physical educator is in this direction. But when the exercise becomes rehabilitative, then it becomes exclusively the function of the physician with technical help from the physical director.

In the final analysis, it is our job as physical educators to get individuals to exercise. The program we organize will dictate how successful we are.

Chapter 5

PROGRAMS OF EXERCISE–
PROGRAM IMPLEMENTATION

WILLIAM C. DAY

In a recent *U. S. News and World Report* article (2), a physician took a rather critical look at jogging as a fitness activity. Along with questioning the prudence of jogging as an activity for the masses, he seemed to fear most the uncontrolled approach to exercise where there is neither medical evaluation nor supervision of the individual. I think many of us share this particular concern.

If adult men are to exercise, the safest and possibly most effective way is through participation in a carefully planned and supervised program of medical evaluation, fitness testing, and conditioning. The content of such a program is the subject of this book. In the next few pages, I would like to share some thoughts on how such a program can be implemented in an organization, such as the YMCA, or as part of larger community programs, such as adult education or city and town recreation.

The following ideas and suggestions are by no means the final solution to the problem of operating a successful physical fitness program. They are the result of some experience in administering a program and the observing of several apparently successful operations in various parts of this country. One of the underlying assumptions is that the participants will be so-called normal, nonpathologic individuals. Programs for the cardiac will be discussed later.

LEADERSHIP

The success of any venture lies ultimately with those who administer and give direction to it. The importance of good professional leadership has already been discussed and cannot be overstressed.

In addition to the capable professional, I would like to consider

[70]

the involvement of a group of individuals who can offer great strength and diversity to an organization's efforts in the area of physical fitness. In YMCA terminology, these are laymen or volunteer leaders. In many cases they are business or professional men, highly intelligent and active members of the community. In *all* cases, they are individuals with a keen interest in physical fitness and/or the sponsoring organization.

No physical educator whom I know has the time or all of the talents and skills necessary to run, by himself, a "first class" physical fitness program. However, there are, in every community, many individuals who, once interested, would contribute their time and particular talents to insure the success of the total program. There are those of us who feel that the ultimate success, or failure, of reaching a significant portion of the population rests with our ability to interest, recruit, and train large numbers of these men who can perform the many tasks which are part of a successful operation.

If there is already a physical fitness program operating in your organization, the search for leadership is relatively easy. Many of those now participating are potential leaders. For those of you who are in the planning stages, it will be somewhat more difficult, but with a little searching, you should find that your community has many individuals who would be delighted to be part of this effort.

One reason, which is sometimes overlooked, for utilizing laymen is that this offers an opportunity for people to become "involved." When people are involved in something, their interest is much keener. The success of anything is also much more likely if large numbers of people become involved in its operation.

FUNCTIONS OF LAY LEADERSHIP

I'd like, next, to consider the functions of this group. There are several important roles which can be filled by the layman.

One of the main roles might be that of serving in an advisory capacity. There is usually an advisory group or committee which makes policies and gives direction to program. It is a wise, if not essential idea to have the medical profession well represented on such a committee. We have also felt that it was helpful to have a lawyer as part of this group. The remainder of this advisory or policy-making body should be made up of interested persons whom you feel will be effective in this role.

Other areas in which the layman might serve are those of test administration and conditioning class leadership. While the medical testing will be primarily in the hands of the MD's with the possible assistance of the physical educator, some of the other testing may be capably handled by the layman serving as the technician. This frees the physical educator for his important role of administering the total operation or possibly for testing which requires more background than the layman may be able to attain.

The volunteer leader has had, in some programs, still other functions. Some of these include the administration of motivational programs such as one-hundred-mile jogging clubs, serving on subcommittees for special events, the processing of test results, and if not actually leading, assisting in conditioning classes. The last item, assisting in classes, might involve observing members of the class for signs of distress, for checking attendance, or for other things of this nature.

TRAINING LAY LEADERSHIP

One of the great mistakes that many of us have made is that of spending far too little time training this important group of people. We give them a little background and then turn them loose to administer a test or lead a class.

While it is difficult to commit already busy people to a great deal of time in classroom or practicum type sessions, it is essential that some of this be done if these men are to be effective.

The layman involved in testing should be given some background in the reasons for testing, what the tests measure and what they do not measure, and he should be competent enough to administer reliably that test to which he is assigned. The class leader should be given some basic information in kinesiology and exercise physiology so that, when he is quizzed by a class member, he does not present him with false information. This will also give him an understanding of why certain exercises are desirable and others are not. In addition, some time should be spent on leadership techniques and actual practice in leading a class. Finally, it is a wise idea to train thoroughly all of your leaders in emergency procedures. This should go beyond just telling them where the phone is located so that help can be called.

Since it can be easily done, do not take these men for granted. With a little imagination, several ways of recognizing their efforts can be devised. It may include a gallery of photographs so that other members of the program will know them and recognize them as leaders. It may be a special dinner with some token of appreciation being presented. Whatever it may be, a little recognition for a job well done goes a long, long way.

RECRUITING PARTICIPANTS

Now that we have dealt with leadership, we are ready to begin looking for participants. I do not know of any ideal way to recruit members. Most of us who have been involved with these types of programs would probably agree that, after a while, the members sell it for you. If you run a sound, well administered, safe operation, this is the best piece of public relations you can have.

However, it takes time to build a program to this point. Therefore, a well planned effort to inform the public is highly desirable.

One of the first principles that should govern any public information program is that care be taken to present sound, scientifically acceptable information. It is easy for us, in the position of a YMCA physical director, health club director, and the like, to fall prey to misinformation, especially that with a dramatic and sensational quality to it. Unfortunately we are besieged with it constantly. Fortunately, on the other hand, the gap between us and the researcher and us and the medical doctor is closing, and there is now less excuse for presenting misinformation to our prospective participants.

As a first step in informing the public, I might suggest that you brush up on your public speaking skills and make it known to local service clubs, private organizations, and church and civic groups that you have an interesting worthwhile message for them.

Prior to this, it would be helpful if you, with the help of a good public relations or advertising man, prepared an attractive, informative brochure. (Incidentally, here is another way to involve a laymen.) Do not try to write a book! Merely present a few facts pertinent to physical fitness and health, a few pictures and the details on how a person gets involved. Then, armed with brochures, you can leave something with the audience once you have completed your presentation.

Radio, television, and newspaper coverage is, of course, a great way to get your message to the public. I know that a YMCA in a neighboring state has a series of spot announcements which are released to local radio stations from time to time, plugging its program. The currently popular interview or "talk" shows are sometimes interested in featuring physical fitness as a topic, and there might be an opportunity, with a little salesmanship, to be a guest on one of these. Incidentally, it would not hurt to make an effort to interest members of these media in participating in your program. If help is needed in your program, there is nothing like dealing with a person who knows what it is all about because he himself is part of it.

Not being an expert in advertising or public relations, let me close this part of the discussion with two more points. Using whatever means are adopted for projecting your message to the public.

(1) *Do not make false claims for your program.* For example, do not tell people they will surely never have a heart attack and will live one hundred years if they are physically fit. This is one way to alienate the medical profession in your community, and it also makes it pretty difficult to explain the first heart attack that occurs to someone who may have been active in your program.

(2) *Speak the public's language.* Be careful of becoming too technical in your terminology. What may be perfectly clear to you because of your background, probably does not mean a thing to an audience not made up of fellow professionals.

PREREQUISITES FOR PARTICIPATION

Now that the leadership spots have been filled and the public is aware of the program, we come to the task of handling prospective participants.

One of the first items is the development of an effective system of handling inquires into the program. This should be done courteously and efficiently. A simple system of record keeping can be devised so that all transactions between your office and the prospective member are recorded. It is poor public relations to have someone show up for testing who is not on your list of registrants and who may have just been a victim of poor record keeping on the part of your office.

Once the individual has indicated an interest, there are a few steps which should preceed actual participation.

First, it is a good idea, if time permits, to have a preliminary interview with the person. This can serve as an opportunity to get to know the person and to explain more thoroughly the program and give him a chance to have his questions answered.

Second, if he is still interested, he should be medically cleared for participation. The extent of this procedure may range from a signed statement from the man's physician to thorough medical testing and evaluation as part of the total testing procedure. The former will more often be the case, in the type of program being discussed in this presentation.

Third, if he has been cleared up to this point, some evaluation of his physical fitness can be made. This might include work capacity tests, evaluation of body composition, tests of flexibility, strength, and any other areas which are considered of interest or importance.

It is at this point where effective use of laymen can be made. Rather than one individual doing all of the testing, several well-trained individuals are involved. This means that it is possible to test groups of individuals in a given time period rather than just one person.

Fourth, after the completion of testing, some of us have held a meeting of all those tested. It may be a luncheon meeting, if the testing is done in the morning. The purpose of this is to:

(1) Enable new members to meet each other before the conditioning program gets underway.

(2) Discuss, generally, the test results and what they mean.

(3) Present the "facts of physical fitness" in an interesting and enlightening way. The use but not the overuse of audio visual material is encouraged.

(4) Explain the details of how the group conditioning program

will be handled and stress the importance of regular attendance and not overdoing.

(5) Answer, if possible, any questions which may arise.

As one more step before workouts begin, an individual meeting with each man is held to deal with specific problems. Here is where limitations are spelled out, and a more detailed discussion of the man's test results may be given.

For example, if your program features jogging, and the man, because of some orthopedic difficulty, is unable to jog, an individualized program of bicycling or swimming may be outlined for him. Many of the extremely unfit men may be asked to participate in a walking program, rather than jogging.

If all is well at this point, the man is ready to participate in the conditioning program.

EDUCATION OF THE PARTICIPANT

It is important, I think, to emphasize that participation should be an educational experience for the individual as well as a means of his relaxing and becoming fit. There are several ways in which he can be educated. A few will be discussed here.

The testing phase, together with group and individual meetings, can be an excellent educational experience if enough good sound preparation goes into them. However, it should not end there.

Effective use can be made of the time immediately before or after a conditioning class for discussion of some aspect of physical fitness. It may, for example, be on the dangers of overstress, the importance of regular participation or the problems of exercising in the heat. Regular discussions of these and other topics are one way of preventing members from developing misconceptions. For example, too many people still are convinced that the only way to lose weight through exercise is to wear a rubber sweat suit.

A well edited newsletter, once in a while, is a good way of keeping people informed of current thinking in this area as well as letting them know some of the newsy things happening to individuals or to the program itself.

Finally, since physical fitness can only be considered one part of a person's total health maintenance, it would be desirable to include education in related areas such as nutrition, smoking, etc. Special sessions, such as a postworkout luncheon or dinner with a guest speaker who is an expert in one of these areas is one way of accomplishing this. One YMCA held a couple of successful Saturday morning breakfast meetings, believe it or not. One was on nutrition; the other, on heart disease and exercise.

MOTIVATING THE PARTICIPANT

Even though we may have done a good job to this point, the task of keeping people motivated is still going to be a problem.

Of course, good leadership and a well run operation are important first steps in accomplishing this. However, some other factors may also be considered.

According to a report given by Dr. Fred Heinzelmann (1) at a recent St. Louis meeting, peoples' motivations for participating change after they are involved for awhile. While they may be initially motivated by fear of heart disease, not feeling as young as they did a few years ago, and reasons like this, the two most important factors which seemed to keep them involved were the quality of leadership and the social aspects of group participation. Neglect of these two factors could mean mediocrity for your program.

Another motivational tool is the reevaluation of the person's fitness once he has been exercising regularly for a few months. Few people are unaffected by seeing objective improvement in their fitness, although with many of them the fact they feel better has already told them that they must have improved.

Many programs around the country have some kind of an award system as a means of motivation. This may take the form of a one-hundred-mile or fifty-mile club where members receive awards for jogging or swimming certain distances. These are fine if steps are taken to prevent an individual from overdoing for the sake of an award or the satisfaction of one's ego. This can be accomplished by limiting the distance for which one can receive credit within a given time period. A further step would be to keep beginning members out of this type of program. Competition should be played down as much as possible.

With a little imagination, other criterion for awards can be devised. Regularity of participation might be another way of recognizing an individual.

While it may seem unimportant to some of you, a tie tack, key chain, or paper weight signifying some level of achievement by the person seems to mean a great deal to him. If wisely used, it can be a worthwhile addition to the total program.

SUMMARY

I have attempted to offer some practical ideas on program implementation. Let me briefly summarize some of these:

(1) There is a wealth of talented and interested people in your organization or community. Get them "involved." Give them an opportunity to have "a piece of the action."

(2) Be selective in the information dispensed to your leaders, participants, and the general public. Be alert to what is factual and what is false.

(3) A well-organized procedure of handling inquiries and bringing participants into programs is essential. Remember, this is a person's first impression of the program and, if the saying is true, it can be a lasting one.

(4) Continually work to educate participants. It should not cease with the initial orientation and testing.

(5) Methods of keeping people motivated should be developed. The importance of group participation, people exercising together and sharing common complaints as well as the joys of becoming fit, cannot be overemphasized.

(6) No matter what fancy frills may ornament any program you design, success can only come with good, well-trained leadership and a safe, well supervised operation.

REFERENCES

1. Heinzelmann, F.: Factors Influencing Response to Physical Activity Programs and the Effects of Participation on Health Attitudes and Behavior. An address given to N.I.R.A. Annual Conference, June 7, 1969.
2. Johnson, Harry J.: Warning to joggers. *U.S. News and World Report.* August 11, 1969.

Chapter 6

MEDICAL EVALUATION FOR
PHYSICAL EXERCISE PROGRAMS*

WILLIAM B. KANNEL

A s a result of recent publicity pointing out the evils of a sedentary life and extolling the virtues of regular physical exercise and main-tenance of physical fitness, many middle-aged and elderly flabby men have taken up jogging and other forms of unaccustomed physical exertion. Those advocating exercise programs and those managing physical exercise facilities have a clear responsibility to safeguard those who may foolishly undertake a program of exercise without either prior medical evaluation or supervision. Included in the advice to the general public over age forty-five to take more exercise should be a caution that they undertake this under medical supervision. Or-ganized physical exercise facilities should require medical certification concerned with the advisability and nature of the exercise program for each individual. Also, periodic medical evaluation for the de-velopment of undesirable side effects and contraindications as well as progress in achieving defined objectives should be included.

This report is concerned with the nature of this medical evalua-tion. From a medical standpoint a physical exercise program can be regarded as part of physical medicine or physiotherapy and may be conceptualized like any form of therapy. Consideration should be given to the rationale for therapy, indications, contraindications, individualized dosage, side effects, and evaluation of response to therapy. The medical evaluation required must take into account all these elements.

* From the Heart Disease Epidemiology Study, Framingham, Massachusetts, and the National Heart Institute, National Institutes of Health, Public Health Service, United States Department of Health, Education and Welfare, Washing-ton, D.C., 20201.

[79]

RATIONALE

For a long time vigorous physical exertion and hard work were considered detrimental to the health of even robust persons, let alone those with diseased hearts. Attitudes have changed, and it is now believed that regular exercise is a requisite for maintenance of optimal cardiac function. Today it is even believed to make a substantial contribution to the rehabilitation of the cardiac patient formerly routinely restricted to an inactive existence.

It is an established fact that physical fitness and supervised exercise are of importance not only in rehabilitation following injury, but in the prevention of musculoskeletal injury. There is also a suspicion that physical exercise and maintenance of fitness can retard some of the "degenerative" processes so ubiquitous in advanced age.

There are many compelling reasons for advocating physical exercise even though adequate statistics concerned with the effect of regular physical exercise on longevity, general health, and cardiovascular health, in particular, are still lacking. Despite the lack of evidence many physicians have come to regard it as an essential hygienic measure as important as adequate sleep, recreation, mental tranquility, and a balanced diet. Physical activity is essential to maintenance of musculoskeletal integrity, efficient venous drainage of the extremities, and function of the cardiovascular apparatus. It is alleged to be helpful in working off nervous tension, relieving insomnia, and improving sexual potency. There is a good reason to council healthy persons against a sedentary existence. Regardless of age, moderate regular exercise can be recommended for healthy persons. It is of undoubted value in those taking up vigorous sports or arduous employment. Vigorous exercise programs, however, can be dangerous for those who are unaccustomed to it if undertaken too precipitously. As in any other mode of therapy there is a hazard associated with overdose or its use when contraindicated.

Rationale in Cardiovascular Disease

It is not unreasonable to consider whether the transformation of man by modern industrial technology from a physically active to a sedentary creature has exacted a toll in ill-health and increased susceptibility to lethal coronary attacks. There is evidence from many

studies of factors leading to heart attacks that lack of adequate physical exercise is a prominent feature in the background of coronary victims who fail to survive their attacks (1-4). The amount and nature of the physical activity involved is uncertain, but data from Framingham and elsewhere suggests that the amount of exercise required to afford substantial protection is quite modest. In Framingham, a subject's risk of coronary attacks in general was found to be substantially higher in persons with a low physical activity index than in those more active (Fig. 6-1). It is notable that those classed "sedentary" (with a physical activity index of 29 or less) who experienced an excess of lethal coronary attacks were virtually motionless people. A physical activity index score of 24 would be obtained by spending all twenty-four hours of the day in bed (4)!

Despite the appearance of a more striking relation of physical activity to fatal than nonfatal coronary attacks in other studies, case fatality rates in Framingham were not related prospectively to antecedent physical activity status. Other studies however have found a striking relationship to fatal outcome retrospectively (14). Thus,

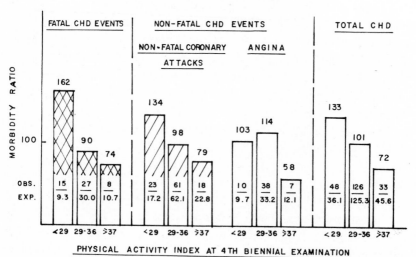

Figure 6-1.

in persons with a compromised coronary circulation it is possible that advice to avoid exercise entirely is not necessarily in the best interest of the potential coronary victim (1-14).

Cardiovascular Effects of Exercise

The mechanism by which physical exercise enhances survival in coronary victims is still a matter of conjecture. Among the hypotheses proposed are improvement in the oxygen economy of the myocardium, development of a more appropriate response of the sympathetic nervous system, transfer of potassium ions into myocardial tissue, and promotion of collateral circulation. It is also possible that some of the beneficial effect of exercise derives from the fact that it brings to light marginal coronary vascular insufficiency at an earlier, more remedial stage by provoking symptoms earlier in the course of the disease. It is not clear how physical exercise can significantly retard the rate of atherogenesis since there is no consistent evidence that exercise produces a sustained lowering of blood lipids in persons on the usual western diet or affects the blood pressure level. Together these appear to be the chief atherogenic precursors of coronary heart disease.

The recognition that physical activity might be beneficial, rather than harmful to the heart, probably had its beginning in the revelation that the enlarged "athlete's heart" was actually a functionally superior pump rather than a liability. Physical exercise and conditioning are known to produce certain beneficial effects on the cardiovascular apparatus. Vigorous exercise can "train" the myocardium so that it hypertrophies and the heart rate slows as each beat becomes more powerful and capable of pumping a greater volume of blood. It is not clear what effect this improvement in the capacity of the myocardium to cope efficiently with a heavy work load has on the pathologic consequences of atherosclerosis. It has been hypothesized that an improvement in the oxygen economy of the heart occurs so it can compensate for a compromised coronary circulation or limit the damage when an occlusion occurs. There is also some evidence that exercise increases the caliber of the coronary arterial circulation both in animals and in man (5, 6). It is not clear, however, whether the size of the coronary arteries per gram of heart

muscle is also improved or whether this can compensate for a local-ized atherothrombotic stenosis. The amount of exercise required to improve either the mechanical efficiency of the heart or the caliber of its vessels is considerable. Since the amount of exercise which appears, from epidemiologic studies of the general population, to be protecting coronary victims from a fatal outcome is quite modest and not intense enough to evoke these effects, another mechanism seems more likely.

More consistent with the epidemiologic data is the hypothesis that exercise promotes collateral circulation to bypass blocked vessels. It has been demonstrated that in animals, whose vessels have been partially blocked, collateral intercommunications between the major coronary arteries can be promoted by exercise and the animals thus protected against the consequences of a myocardial infarction when a total occlusion is subsequently produced (7). Such collaterals can *not* be produced by exercise unless the vessels are at least par-tially blocked (8). A supplementary arterial supply can be demon-strated in the hearts of patients with severe coronary atherosclerosis proportional to the severity of involvement. This can probably be demonstrated even if they do not exercise, since many were too in-capacitated by their disease to tolerate any exercise. A region of ischemic myocardium somehow stimulates the opening of collateral channels, possibly in response to anoxia or increased pressure gradients across the gap between closed and patent vessels. Exercise, which transiently accentuates this process, could promote this corrective opening of collateral channels and their eventual development into a functionally important adjunct to the deficient blood supply, minimizing the possibly disastrous consequences.

INDICATIONS AND CONTRAINDICATIONS
Indications

Many of the indications for exercise programs have been enumer-ated in the discussion of the rationale for exercise. There is much to suggest that properly implemented and supervised endurance types of exercise are a most important contributor to a long and healthy life. To begin with, lack of physical fitness itself may be considered as an indication for physical exercise as may its usual accompaniments of obesity, breathlessness on modest exertion, and a rapid resting pulse rate without other explanation. To recapitulate, physical exercise may be prescribed for a variety of disorders other than simply lack of physical fitness. These include coronary prevention, osteoporosis, low back complaints, senile emphysema, rehabilitation following injury, general musculoskeletal deterioration, rehabilitation of stroke and coronary victims, nervous tension, insomnia, and decreased sexual potency, among others. It is also clearly indicated in those planning once again to take up vigorous sports or an arduous occupation.

Contraindications

While the benefits of physical activity are many, there are distinct potential hazards and some specific contraindications for general, unsupervised exercise programs. Medical assessment for an exercise program must include a consideration of general health and, in particular, identification of specific contraindications to unrestricted exercise. The major contraindications include orthopedic difficulties, chronic respiratory disease, and cardiovascular disorders.

General Physical Condition

General physical condition of the subject or the existence of general medical disorders may constitute at least a temporary contraindication for general exercise programs. Severe anemia, thyroid disorders, insulin-dependent diabetes, and severe hypertension are among those encountered with some frequency. A general medical checkup is wise before undertaking vigorous exercise programs.

Respiratory Disorders

Respiratory disorders in general provide little contraindication except during acute exacerbations. Obstructive emphysema, however, may well constitute a contraindication, particularly the bullous variety. There is the possibility that the condition may be aggravated and pneumothorax precipitated by strenuous exercise. Generally, impaired ventilatory function in emphysematous patients precludes their participation in endurance types of exercise. Rare instances of quiescent pulmonary tuberculosis, sarcoidosis with alveolar-capillary block, restrictive ventilatory defects, severe adhesive pleuritis, and pulmonary fibrosis, pulmonary granulomas and post-thoracotomy surgical chest residues do exist, but such persons seldom present themselves for evaluation for physical exercise programs.

Orthopedic Disorders

Orthopedic disorders deserve careful consideration since unaccustomed exercise places unusual stress on the musculoskeletal apparatus. Active exercise during a flare-up of arthritis, bursitis, tendonitis, or intervertebral disc is not recommended. Even persons without known orthopedic difficulties often develop minor strains, sprains, and joint derangements. Between flare-ups special exercises designed to increase the range of painless motion and to prevent contractures, muscle atrophy, and osteoporosis are considered helpful. However, both excessive exercise and the total lack of it increases discomfort and disability.

Cardiovascular Disorders

Cardiovascular disorders are among the most prominent contraindications for general, unrestricted exercise programs because of the potential lethal consequences. Since the side effects are apt to be catastrophic, especial attention to the cardiovascular status of middle-aged applicants for unaccustomed exercise is mandatory. Each candidate should be examined for a number of overt cardiovascular conditions, including any evidence of impending or recent myocardial infarction, anginal distress, ventricular or aortic aneurysm, aortic stenosis, coarctation and other congenital anomalies, massive or unexplained cardiac enlargement, recent pulmonary embolism, pulmonary hypertension, and excessively high systemic blood pressure. Minor valvular deformity manifested only by heart murmurs, but without evidence of impaired cardiac function or specific chamber enlargement, need not be a contraindication for an exercise program and supervised exercise may actually be helpful.

In addition to these overt evidences of cardiovascular disease, certain findings of occult disease, even in completely asymptomatic persons, may represent a contraindication for an unsupervised general exercise program although such persons may well benefit from less vigorous, controlled exercise. A lack of cardiac symptoms or physical findings in a middle-aged male is no guarantee that all is well since advanced coronary artery disease can and does exist in persons who believe themselves to be in good health. Persons who are highly vulnerable to CHD, or who have already acquired it in an occult form, are quite common in the general population. Actual myocardial infarctions may be found on ECG examination in persons who had no recognized cardiovascular complaints. In fact, at Framingham where routine biennial ECG surveillance of the population has been maintained for twenty years, one in every five documented myocardial infarctions was silent or unrecognized (Fig. 6-2). Furthermore, unheralded, sudden, unexpected death may be the first mani-

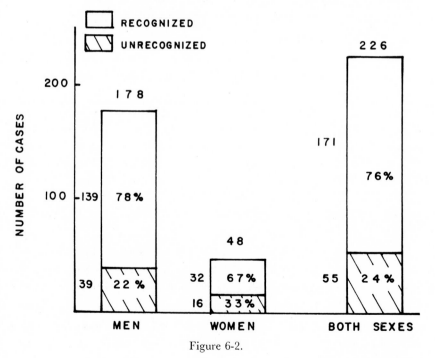

PROPORTION OF ECG-DOCUMENTED MYOCARDIAL INFARCTIONS UNRECOGNIZED (16 YEARS) MEN AND WOMEN 30-62 AT ENTRY: FRAMINGHAM STUDY

Figure 6-2.

festation of coronary disease in persons who believe themselves in good health. Fully 65 percent of all deaths during coronary attacks are sudden and unexpected, the whole course of the illness lasting a matter of minutes. In fact, one in six coronary attacks presents with sudden death as the first and only manifestation. Even symptomatic heart attacks from which persons have survived characteristically struck without warning in persons believed to be well. However, such persons were seldom free of stigmata which could have forewarned of the impending disaster. Since potential victims of coronary attacks are usually entirely asymptomatic and have little reason to question their health, they must be routinely examined for certain hallmarks of increased vulnerability to coronary disease, advanced coronary stenosis, and occult coronary heart disease.

This can be readily accomplished economically and without trauma to the subject by the physician employing ordinary office procedures and simple laboratory tests. Existing coronary heart disease can be excluded by a history for angina, myocardial infarction, and a current electrocardiogram. Unrecognized infarctions can be uncovered in this way, as can others less certain, but highly suspicious indicators of coronary heart disease in the resting electrocardiogram. Persons with electrocardiographic left ventricular hypertrophy have been shown to develop a distinct excess of symptomatic coronary attacks and death, no less often than those with actual myocardial infarction (15). Persons with intraventricular block have also been shown to have an increased risk of coronary events (9). It would seem unjustified to submit such persons to unrestricted exercise programs. Still earlier evidence of a compromised coronary circulation can be obtained by an electrocardiogram secured after a standard exercise test. Changes provoked by exercise, even in robust young men, have been shown prospectively to be associated with a marked excess development of coronary attacks (10, 13).

Highly vulnerable persons who have not yet progressed to this stage may also be identified with relative ease. These hallmarks of vulnerability have been gleaned from an examination of the characteristics of persons who have gone on to develop coronary disease in comparison to their cohorts in Framingham who have remained free of it over sixteen years of observation. Using the values of a number of readily ascertained medical attributes, a logistic risk function can be computed for each person making it possible to place asymptomatic persons into categories according to their probability of having a coronary attack over a thirtyfold range of risks (Table 6-I). Thus, persons who had "atherogenic" traits, such as hypertension, elevated cholesterol levels, or ECG abnormalities, developed a distinct excess

TABLE 6-I

TWELVE-YEAR INCIDENCE OF CHD
ACCORDING TO DECILE OF RISK

Decile of Risk*	2187 Men Obs. Cases	Observed 12-Year Incid/1000	2669 Women Obs. Cases	Observed 12-Year Incid/1000
10	82	375	54	202
9	44	201	23	86
8	31	142	21	79
7	33	151		52
6	22	101	5	19
5	20	91	6	22
4	15	59	2	7
3	10	46	0	0
2	3	14	3	11
1	0	0	1	4
Total	258	118	129	48

*Deciles of Risk According to: age, SBP, rel. wt., Hb., no. cigs. Level of all of following—ECG ABN., Chol. (Using Multiple Logistic Function)

of coronary heart disease, and the risk increased with the number of these and other risk factors that were present (15). Persons with one or more of these traits must be considered highly vulnerable and liable to have accelerated coronary artery atherosclerosis. Their probability of having asymptomatic advanced coronary artery disease is considerably greater than that of the general population. While there is evidence to suggest that such persons may benefit from a supervised exercise program, there is justified fear that unrestricted vigorous exercise could prove lethal. Specially designed and supervised exercise programs could be quite beneficial for such persons by promoting collateral circulation. Such vulnerable persons can prudently be encouraged to take some form of supervised exercise rather than being restricted to a sedentary existence. It is conceivable that in persons vulnerable to coronary atherosclerosis, advice to avoid exercise entirely may actually condemn them to a fatal outcome when their coronary attack occurs.

In all these recommendations it must be recognized that the same ischemic stimulus to collateral development may also provoke necrosis of the myocardium. Thus, promotion of collaterals by exercise may be beneficial but only providing it does not, in the process, provoke a coronary attack instead. Hence, caution is essential in implementing exercise programs in persons likely to have advanced coronary sclerosis, symptomatic or not.

One real fear that plagues those recommending and supervising physical exercise programs in flabby middle-aged men or known cardiacs is the possible catastrophic occurrence of sudden collapse and death while exercising. As indicated in the foregoing, the ischemia provoked by exercise is a double-edged sword which may also provoke ventricular fibrillation. Data from Framingham suggests that persons with one or more coronary risk factors, i.e. the cigarette habit, ECG abnormalties, and multiple atherogenic traits, are particularly prone to sudden unexpected death (Fig. 6-3). Persons with "sedentary traits," most in need of exercise, are also more liable to sudden unexpected death (Fig. 6-4). Whether reflecting sedentary status or something else, persons with a rapid resting pulse rate or

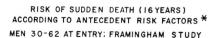

RISK OF SUDDEN DEATH (16 YEARS)
ACCORDING TO ANTECEDENT RISK FACTORS *
MEN 30-62 AT ENTRY: FRAMINGHAM STUDY

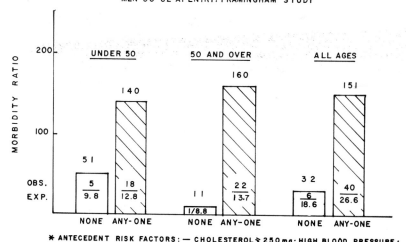

* ANTECEDENT RISK FACTORS: — CHOLESTEROL ≯ 250 mg; HIGH BLOOD PRESSURE; ECG ABNORMALITY; DIABETES; CIGARETTES ˃ 1 PKG./DAY

Figure 6.3

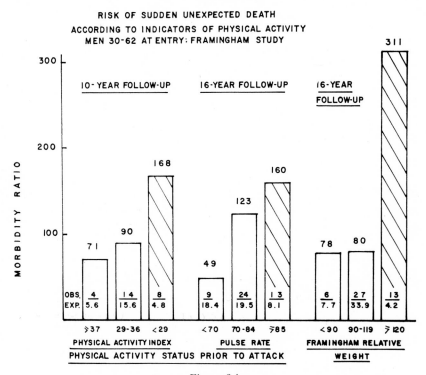

RISK OF SUDDEN UNEXPECTED DEATH
ACCORDING TO INDICATORS OF PHYSICAL ACTIVITY
MEN 30-62 AT ENTRY: FRAMINGHAM STUDY

Figure 6.4

who were obese had an increased propensity to fatal coronary attacks, and the risk mounted precipitously in those with the combination of these traits (Fig. 6-5). It would seem prudent that such persons be induced gradually, stopped short of vigorous peak load or endurance exercise, not allowed competitive sports, and allowed a period of defervescence after exercise.

MEDICAL EVALUATION

Taking all of the foregoing into consideration, the problem of the nature of the medical evaluation required can be addressed. To be practical, the evaluation must be economical, atraumatic, and efficient, employing equipment and procedures readily available to the practicing physician. Since the state of knowledge is regrettably incomplete, acceptable guidelines of proven value do not exist. We must at the present time dwell in the realm of the probable.

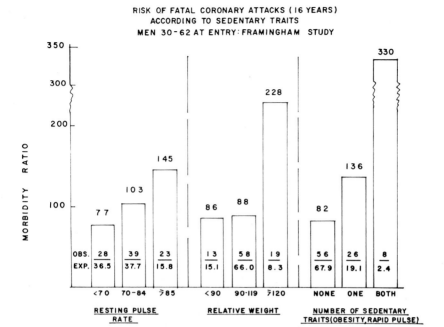

Figure 6.5

It is wise to begin with a *general medical assessment* unless the subject is well known to the examiner and has been under periodic medical surveillance. This is designed to uncover occult medical conditions which should be corrected prior to undertaking an exercise program. A careful review of organ symptoms, a past history of illness, a general physical examination, and a number of laboratory tests should be obtained routinely. Thus, conditions such as anemia, latent diabetes, or asymptomatic hypertension may be uncovered.

The general medical assessment should include an assessment of physical fitness. Unless specifically looked for, physical deterioration because of lack of exercise can be missed in the usual physical examination. Evaluation of living habits and alteration in physical appearance or function will usually provide indications of physical deterioration. These signs include accumulation of abdominal fat, loss of muscle strength and endurance, a decrease in cardiorespiratory efficiency, loss of musculoskeletal flexibility, breathlessness on moderate exertion, slowed reaction time, and impaired balance. The physical fitness assessment should therefore include simple office procedures, such as weighing the patient, measuring skinfold thickness with Lange calipers, dynamometry to test muscle strength, and a total vital capacity. These can be readily carried out by an office nurse. Physical examination, taking note of a rapid pulse rate, musculoskeletal inflexibility of the back and shoulders, poor posture with chin and chest dropped and abdomen protruding, graphically tells the story denoting poor physical condition.

Unless explained by some other cause, or by excitement or apprehension, pulse rates between seventy-six and eighty-six per minute may reflect poor physical fitness. Those above eighty-six at rest usually reflect either apprehension or medical pathology. Lower pulse rates generally denote good physical condition, and a well trained athlete will have a rate in the fifties.

Most physicians do not have the time, training, or equipment to employ the sophisticated methods available to the work physiologist for the purpose of assessing fitness. Evaluation of cardiac function and maximum oxygen uptake have come to be accepted as the best yardstick in judging fitness. Pulse rate in response to exercise is a convenient indicator feasible in clinical practice. A number of dynamic tests of fitness based on changes in pulse rates in response to an exercise load are applicable in a clinical situation. Two of these are the Harvard Step Test and the Cooper 1.5-mile test. These agree reasonably well with optimal assessments of the capacity of the cardiovascular and respiratory system to deliver oxygen to the musculoskeletal apparatus as measured by maximum oxygen uptakes.

Most investigators agree that men can be allowed to participate in a vigorous physical activity program if they manifest no difficulties with exertion sufficient to raise their pulse rate to 170 in their twenties and 10 beats per minute under this for each successive decade in age. It is safe to allow a moderately intense physical exercise program in the absence of evidence of physical stress or abnormality in the electrocardiogram under either a step, bicycle, or treadmill exercise test load sufficient to raise the heart rate to the above levels.

It might be argued that an adequate assessment for a vigorous exercise program requires physiologic testing under physical work loads at least equivalent to that which may be encountered in the proposed exercise program. However, even this is no guarantee since susceptibility may vary widely depending on intrinsic or environmental circumstances, such as ambient temperature and humidity, fluid and electrolyte balance, whether a cigarette is smoked, and proximity to a meal, among others. How stringent pre-exercise dynamic testing under induced physical loads should be remains to be determined, probably by a combination of the application of sound physiological principles and in the final analysis experience.

Evaluation of Respiratory Function

Evaluation of respiratory function by means of total vital capacity and expiratory flow rate determination is a useful procedure in evaluation for physical exercise. Emphysema is an insidious disorder which has usually progressed to an advanced stage before the victim is aware of disability. He may at some point wonder if a physical exercise program will "improve his wind," attributing breathlessness to poor physical condition. Spirometry is required to detect less advanced disease that is not revealed by overt physical signs such as hyperresonance, distant breath sounds, prolonged expiration, expiratory wheezing, barrel-shaped chest, and low, flat diaphragms with a restricted excursion. Ideally, a chest x-ray should also be included to check for bullae, heart size, pulmonary vascular engorgement, effusions, and emphysema.

Orthopedic Evaluation

Orthopedic evaluation should include an inspection and palpation of major joints for tenderness, redness, deformity, subcutaneous nodules, subluxation, internal derangement, and effusions. In particular, the range of motion, stability, and flexibility of the weight-bearing joints, including the back, should be tested. Since unaccustomed exercise often provokes minor orthopedic side effects, orthopedic difficulties warrant careful consideration. Even minor impairment, such as postural defects and flat feet, may presage difficulties which may discourage the subject from continuing. Many orthopedic problems which interfere with adherence to exercise programs can be anticipated. Forewarned, their likelihood of so doing can be decreased by proper conditioning.

Cardiovascular Evaluation

Cardiovascular evaluation is perhaps the most essential feature of medical assessment for exercise programs because of the possible catastrophic consequences. Most cardiac contraindications are readily detected on ordinary office physical examination, chest x-ray, and an electrocardiogram. This will detect cardiac murmurs, arrhythmias, an enlarged heart, hypertrophy, intraventricular block, hypertension, congenital anomalies, and signs of myocardial insufficiency.

Since a serious degree of impaired coronary circulation may exist without a single symptom or physical finding, the use of certain biochemical and electrocardiographic tests would appear prudent. An electrocardiogram at rest is required to detect occult disease such as an unrecognized myocardial infarction, left ventricular hypertrophy by electrocardiogram and intraventricular block. Despite their asymptomatic state persons with these findings are highly vulnerable to lethal coronary attacks (9, 15). The survival of those with unrecognized myocardial infarctions is no better than that of those with a history of symptomatic infarctions (Fig. 6-6). While such persons benefit from a carefully supervised restricted program of exercise, vigorous competitive exercise could be disastrous.

In addition to obtaining an electrocardiogram at rest, a postexercise electrocardiogram to detect occult ischemic myocardial impairment in those with atherogenic precursors, such as hypercholesterolemia ($\geqslant$ 260 mg%), hypertension ($\geqslant$ 160/95 mm Hg), and impaired carbohydrate tolerance (2-hr postprandial blood sugar $>$ 160 mg%), is indicated.

Consequently, cardiac evaluation should include in addition to the standard history, physical examination, chest x-ray, and electrocardiogram at rest, and a postexercise electrocardiogram; particularly in those whose blood examination reveals hypercholesterolemia or impaired carbohydrate tolerance, or in whom there is hypertension.

Evaluation for Response to Exercise

A number of investigators have reported improvement in ischemic

SURVIVAL FOLLOWING INITIAL MYOCARDIAL INFARCTION
MEN AND WOMEN 30-79:FRAMINGHAM HEART STUDY

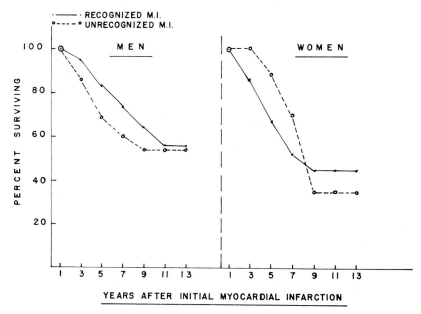

Figure 6.6.

S-T displacement under a work load after training. These ECG changes could result from improved myocardial efficiency, changes in peripheral distribution of blood and its return, decreased flow or pressure requirements, and an increase in coronary vascularization.

Reduction in body weight or flabbiness as indicated by skin-fold thickness and abdominal girth, improvement in musculoskeletal flexibility and pulse rate at rest and in response to an exercise load are useful indicators of a favorable response to an exercise program.

Subjective improvement, including an enhanced feeling of well-being, self-confidence, and work capacity, are to be expected. If instead, sustained breathlessness, exertional chest discomfort, easy fatigability, a persistent musculoskeletal soreness, and pain are encountered, the advisability of continuation should be reconsidered.

COMMENTS

There is a good deal of confusion concerning the merits and hazards of exercise. It is difficult to know whether the net effect of the current enthusiasm for unsupervised exercise will be beneficial or not. There is much to suggest that properly implemented endurance exercise is an important contributor to a long and healthy life.

Better means for assessing physical fitness in the office should be devised. Limited health manpower sufficiently trained and skilled in the disciplines of physical conditioning and therapeutic exercise programs at present prevents optimal supervision of all who need exercise.

Before a sedentary person begins unrestricted exercise, he should have a thorough medical examination to exclude contraindications. This should include orthopedic, respiratory, and cardiovascular evaluation. It should also include an assessment of physical fitness. Since advanced coronary artery disease is not uncommon in persons without either symptoms or physical findings, evaluation for coronary-proneness and occult coronary heart disease should be included. This entails an electrocardiogram at rest and when indicated by hypertension, hypercholesterolemia, or impaired carbohydrate tolerance, a postexercise electrocardiogram.

The minimal amount and type of exercise required to achieve optimal physical fitness and to protect against lethal coronary attacks needs to be better delineated. There is also a need to demonstrate whether or not physical reconditioning after a coronary attack actually reduces the propensity to recurrences and prolongs life. There is evidence that it does help to restore self-confidence and enjoyment of living and that it improves work capacity. The hazards as well as the benefits of carefully supervised postinfarction exercise programs need to be ascertained, but there is much to suggest that the potential benefits far exceed the hazards. More discreet guidelines and criteria are needed to delineate the indications and contraindications and to insure safety and efficacy.

REFERENCES

1. Morris, J. N., Hardy, J. A., Raffle, P. A. B., Roberts, C. G., and Parks, J. W.: Coronary heart disease and physical activity of work. *Lancet,* 2:1053, 1953.
2. Kahn, H. A.: The relationship of reported coronary heart disease mortality to physical activity of work. *Amer J Public Health, 53*:1058, 1963.

3. Taylor, H. L., Klepetar, E., Keys, A., Parlin, W., Blackburn, H., and Puchert, T.: Death rates among physically active and sedentary employees of the railroad industry. *Amer J Public Health, 52*:1697, 1962.
4. Kannel, W. B.: Habitual level of physical activity and risk of coronary heart disease. *Canad Med Ass J, 96*:821, 1967.
5. Stevenson, J. A. F., Feleki, V., Rechnitzer, P., Beaton, J. R.: Effect of exercise on coronary tree size in the rat. *Circ Res, 15*:265, 1964.
6. Tepperman, J., Pearlman, D.: Effects of exercise and anemia on coronary arteries of small animals as revealed by the Corrosion-Cast Technique. *Circ Res, 9*:576-584, 1961.
7. Eckstein, R. W.: Effect of exercise and coronary artery narrowing on coronary collateral circulation. *Circ Res, 5*:230, 1967.
8. Burt, J. S., and Jackson, R.: The effects of physical exercise on the coronary collateral circulation of dogs. *J Sports Med, 5*:203, 1965.
9. Kannel, W. B., Kagan, A., Dawber, T. R., and Revotskie, N.: Epidemiology of coronary heart disease: Implications for the practicing physician. *Geriatrics, 17*:675, October, 1962.
10. Mattingly, T. W.: The post-exercise electrocardiogram. Its value in the diagnosis and prognosis of coronary arterial disease. *Amer J Cardiol, 9*:395, 1962.
11. Rumball, A., and Acheson, E. D.: Latent coronary heart disease detected by electrocardiogram before and after exercise. *Brit Med J.: 5328*:423, 1963.
12. Brody, A. J.: Master two-step exercise test in clinically unselected patients. *JAMA, 171*:1195, 1959.
13. Robb, G. P., and Marks, H. H.: Latent coronary artery disease: Determination of its presence and severity by the exercise electrocardiogram. *Amer J Cardiol, 13*:603, 1964.
14. Shapiro, S., Weinblatt, E., Frank, C. W., and Sager, R. V.: Incidence of Coronary heart disease in a population insured for medical care (HIP). *Amer J Public Health, 59 (suppl, part II)*: 1-101, 1969.
15. Kannel, W. B., Gordon, T., and Offutt, D.: Left ventricular hypertrophy by electrocardiogram. Prevalence, incidence and mortality in the Framingham Study. *Ann Int Med, 71*:89-105, 1967.

Chapter 7

LEGAL ASPECTS OF EXERCISE PROGRAMS

STACY H. DOBRZENSKY

THE legal concepts involved are not complicated—factual questions pose the major problems. Perhaps this overview of the legal aspects will set the stage for discussion of particular situations of concern.

Let us assume that, on the basis of a staff suggestion, the idea of a joint effort for putting on an exercise program is developed and presented to the local Heart and Y Boards, which authorize a joint committee to carry out a plan to (a) develop guidelines for exercise programs, (b) plan and undertake programs for training individuals in physical fitness and exercise (for-do-it-yourselfers), and (c) plan and undertake physical fitness and exercise classes at the YMCA.

Let us deal with (c), the exercise classes.

The Heart Association and the Y, in a series of meetings and conferences (a) enlist a well-known high school coach and a local cardiologist intensely interested in the concept of exercise and (b) arrange for regular use of the YMCA gym, (c) physical trainers, (d) publicity, and (e) an application form which requires the applicant to certify that he will have consulted his physician to ascertain the propriety of his undertaking the course, described as moderate to periodically strenuous exercise over a stated period and frequency and to certify that he acknowledges that the program is provided by Heart and the Y as voluntary, charitable organizations and that the applicant assumes any risk of injury or death and waives any claim for damages for injury to person or property.

Client No. 1 is twenty-seven years of age, male, married with four children, an electronics engineer with a promising future with a major electrical equipment manufacturer. Client No. 2 is forty years of age, a CPA, the tax partner in a leading national CPA firm, a bachelor.

Client No. 1's wife has called me to say that her husband suffered a severe cardiovascular accident during a session of the class, is in the hospital, and is severely paralyzed with little hope of rehabilitation or return to other than simple, routine work performed at home.

Later, Client No. 2, who knows me because we have a mutual client, calls me from the local hospital to tell me that he slipped and fell when he stepped on a broken stair tile on leaving the exercise class in which he participated, broke his leg, and will be out of action for three or four months, and it is during tax season and what should he do.

First of all, we are concerned with the amount of time that one has within which to file a lawsuit, if one is to be filed, that is, within the statute of limitations. The general rule gives one year within which to file an action for personal injury, two years for property damage. After that time, the action is barred. This does not mean the case has to be finished; simply it has to be commenced by the filing of a complaint.

The next thing we discuss is, "Who do we sue?" Who do we join or make parties to our lawsuit?

We must join every party necessary to a complete determination of the issues of the case. Of perhaps equal importance is the fact one rarely knows which of the defendants has funds sufficient to satisfy any judgment or is covered by insurance. It is most distressing to win a lawsuit only to find that the party against whom you have a judgment is unable to respond financially!

We join the Heart Association and the Y because they furnish the program and the YMCA facilities, the coach because of his role in setting up the specific exercises that were employed, the trainer who conducted the class on the night in question, the physician who advised the committee and approved the scheduling and content of the classes, and Client No. 1's physician and others having significant roles in the program or control of the Y's facilities. If either client's injury had been aggravated at some point following the incidents directly involved, we would have to consider additional defendants.

In the case of the accountant, our primary target is the Y since his injury resulted from the condition of the stairs, but we join the Heart Association as a joint sponsor of the program that made use of the Y building.

Going back to the young cardiovascular victim, he had seen his physician as suggested in the application form and had been given a clean bill of health, in fact, was told he should "tear into this exercise business, you should get in shape and stay in shape—don't over-do it of course!" So we must consider whether to join the physician as a defendant, the theory for which would be negligence (which means carelessness) in the conduct of the checkup and the giving of advice in anticipation of the exercise program, using as a standard the level of medical training, knowledge, and skill prevailing in the area.

Now, what are the rules of the road? For those of you who have already taken the course in "torts," you will hear nothing new and find that I will have highly simplified the subject.

Very briefly, a tort is a private, civil wrong not founded upon contract. It is distinguished from a crime in that, in tort, the law gives the individual a remedy against the wrong doer; in crimes the state steps in to punish the wrongdoer.

Torts divide themselves into three basic categories: (a) intentional wrongs, (b) liability without regard to fault (as when one stores dynamite in his basement in a residential neighborhood), and (c) "negligence" or "unintended harm." Negligence can consist of a careless act or a careless failure to act. There are basically five "earmarks" of liability for unintended wrongs. First, we have to find a "duty of care;" thus, the Y has the duty to maintain its stairways in a safe condition; we have to choose instructors reasonably qualified for the particular task; we have to devise the physical exercise with due regard for the participants we might expect to attend.

Given this "duty of care," we ask if there was a "breach" of that duty. Did we do, or fail to do, something? Did the Y fail reasonably to check its stairways and their condition of repair; did we choose unskilled persons for jobs requiring a degree of skill? It should be noted that the mere existence of a duty of care and of some injury does not necessarily mean that the duty of care was breached. Thus, if we had a safely maintained set of stairs and one visitor dropped a banana skin on the way in, and the next visitor, two minutes later, stepped on it, we could not say that the management had breached its duty of care to members of the public using the facility, for lack of reasonable opportunity to learn of the banana skin, and to remove it.

The next item is what we call "proximate cause," or legal cause. Was the act, that allegedly breached the duty of care, the direct and proximate cause of the injury that ensued. In other words, the act or neglect must have caused the harm in a reasonably direct chain of circumstances.

The fourth item is called "legal harm." Did something that the law protects one from occur? The mere doing of a careless act, or failing to act, where no one is affected, produces no "legal harm." Thus, if my Client No. 2 stepped on a broken tile but was able to take the next step with no more consequence than for the broken tile to fall behind him, he would not have suffered "legal harm."

The last item is usually tied in pretty closely with the previous one. Some damage or injury must have resulted. Thus, in my illustration of the loose tile, if the man had fallen but without injuring himself, we might expect an award of damages of one dollar, simply to recognize the invasion of his legal right.

At this point I might mention that money damages are a poor substitute for a broken leg or a heart attack, or other injury, but you must note that money is all that the law has to use for restitution. We have not yet devised a way to erase or unbreak a broken leg, etc.

Also on the subject of damages, there are basically three types, "special damages," like lost wages, hospital and doctor's bills necessarily incurred for treatment as a result of the injury; "general damages" is the amount of money awarded for pain, suffering, humiliation, etc., that are not reflected in the loss of payment of specified sums as in the case of hospital and ambulance bills. The third category is called "punitive damages," usually not easy to obtain and reserved for cases of vicious or grossly negligent conduct, or fraud.

A question oftentimes asked has to do with the liability of a charitable organization. Charitable funds, corporations, etc. generally are liable for wrongs committed by their officers, agents, and employees. Those jurisdictions where charitable corporations are not liable for torts are behind the times, and it would be most unwise to rely on any such immunity. In any event, the individual who actually committed the negligent act, or omission, would be liable for his own wrong whether or not his association was liable.

Another frequently asked question has to do with liability of board members. The general rule is that a member of the board, as such, is not liable for the consequences of his acts if he acted in good faith and exercised his discretion rather than acted arbitrarily or capriciously. In other words, the board must consider matters and pass judgment upon the basis of a reasonably complete set of facts. The exception, of course, would be the individual who himself was responsible for a wrongful act or omission to act, as where an officer of an association, while on association business, negligently collides his car with that of another, or where he assumes some role in the exercise program and does it negligently.

I might also mention that two can be liable where negligent acts or omission concur in producing the harm. Thus, both Heart and the Y may be held, and where a man is injured on a defective stair and later an ambulance attendant aggravates the injury, both would be liable.

Next, we can consider the defenses to actions. There are two that are probably already in your minds, the "assumption of risk" and the "waiver of any claim." There is one other, that of "contributory negligence." If the party aggrieved *himself* was guilty of negligence, then he may not recover. Of interest is the fact that maritime law applies the doctrine of "comparative negligence." When two ships collide, we measure the degree of negligence of each vessel and apportion the damage between them.

On the subject of the "assumption of risk," naturally we all assume some risk, just by getting up in the morning, or by coming to a Heart Association Symposium. Some occurrence might result in harm. Generally, one is deemed to assume the ordinary risks of enterprises that he undertakes voluntarily. A document to the effect that one assumes the risk of injury to person or property extends only to those dangers of which one has knowledge and only as to ordinary risks. One is entitled to assume that the proprietor of a building will maintain it without negligence, but not that an object will have been dropped on a stair. While it is not generally the policy of the law to exempt one from liability for the consequences of his own wrong, "waivers" may relate to ordinary negligence, but not to fraud, willful conduct, willful injury, or violation of law. Whether or not the assumption of risk or the waiver of damages is a good defense to an action of this kind depends upon the circumstances of the particular case. Having such a provision in an application or contract is certainly no substitute for the exercise of reasonable care.

You will have noticed the word "reasonable" at a number of points in my remarks, or in other connections. This whole subject of negligence, or of torts, is bound up with the concept of the "reasonable and prudent man." We ask ourselves, in judging a tort's question, "Could a reasonable and prudent person in the same circumstances be reasonably expected to have foreseen the kind of harm that occurred in this case?"

At this point your program makes note of the "argument to the jury." That part of a jury trial at which counsel for the plaintiff gives his opening argument, the defendant's counsel gives his argument, and then the plaintiff (probably having held back his choicest morsels) gives the closing argument is a most interesting and stimulating (and often times nerve-wracking) experience. I will not indulge you, however, with one of my finer efforts along these lines; instead let me mention briefly the "persuasion" part of the case. That is, in the "weaving together of fact and law, to state the plaintiff's case," we naturally try to present the clearest, the strongest case for our position. It is important to look at a set of facts, or to look at a set of possible facts, in planning such things as exercise programs as though presented by an adverse party with "dollar signs in his eyes" and "out for blood." To evaluate a situation otherwise is, in my judgment, negligence.

I find that it is often overlooked that the attorney who presents his client's case is not the same person that you might have joined for lunch or sat with at a Board meeting. At the times that he is preparing and presenting the case and arguing to the jury, he is the plaintiff; he is expressing the plaintiff's wishes, desires, hopes, and fears, adding to the plaintiff's own personal qualities, the lawyer's legal talent. I emphasize that he is not the same person you may know socially, whom you might expect to be most sympathetic to the good work that your organization does; he is the plaintiff. He may seem callous in his regard for the parties and witnesses on the other side; he will not be looking for your better side, your high purposes. He will be trying, as the saying goes, to "shoot you down" simply because our aggrieved plaintiffs are seeking recompense from you for damages they believe you caused or are responsible for.

Therefore, in evaluating your legal "risk factors," be sure that your people do not take the position that the "Heart Association" or the Y are "charitable organizations, doing public good; our volunteers are leading citizens; no one will look at things *that* way." Look through the eyes of plaintiff's counsel instead.

And a word about insurance—(a) Obtain it with the help of an experienced broker, not just any salesman you happen to know. (b) Be sure your coverage is broad enough and in high enough limits. (c) Be certain the premiums are paid when due. (d) Consult your broker about the new exercise program, see if you are covered and whether or not you have high enough limits. If he says you are covered, it will not hurt to send him a confirming letter, just in case he is wrong. It is also important to note that your insurance company will provide the lawyers to defend the case, if one should develop, even if the plaintiff fails to recover.

On the question of possible improvements in the law, by and large you will always be exposed to litigation and liability, and I see no particularly useful purpose to be served by Heart Associations or the Y doing more than to alert their advisory committee of their concerns. This is not to say that it is not worthwhile to consider the state of the law and the possibility of change.

You may well ask about possible extensions of the so-called good samaritan laws. California recently enacted, and our Governor signed, a bill that would excuse from liability hospital rescue teams that respond to emergencies. Even with the new law, there are two wide open questions that can be the subject of litigation; first, whether there was truly an emergency, and secondly, whether the hospital exercised proper care in selecting, training, equipping, assigning, and otherwise instructing the members of the team.

One closing note concerning your use of the services of attorneys in connection with specific situations. It has been my experience that but a few understand what it is that an attorney undertakes, the commitment that he in effect makes, when he furnishes you with a legal opinion. An opinion regarding a proposed course of action, if incorrect, may expose the attorney to liability. In a case involving large sums, he has assumed an equally large responsibility. It is the responsibility so assumed that is an important factor in fee setting. Few lawyers can afford to assume such responsibility without charge, although they are free to, and many times do offer to act without compensation.

Chapter 8

PHYSICAL TRAINING AND CORONARY HEART DISEASE*

EUGENE Z. HIRSCH, HERMAN K. HELLERSTEIN
AND CATHEL A. MACLEOD

INTRODUCTION

IN RECENT years much research has been concerned with the feasibility and possible benefits of physical reconditioning of the coronary subject (1-16). A good deal of this research has of necessity been concerned with determining the validity of methods of treatment widely practiced during the first half of the century. The tenets of this therapy required the physician to prescribe prolonged bed rest for the coronary patient and the adoption of a new mode of restrictive living, having as its major components the abrogation of responsibility and a general avoidance of all "stress." The results of this approach frequently caused young coronary subjects to interrupt permanently their active lives, substituting physical and intellectual inactivity and promoting an atmosphere of helplessness with the fear of ever-impending death. Lack of knowledge at that time made an extremely conservative medical attitude necessary. It has become apparent that the natural course of coronary artery disease was not improved by such therapy.

Following World War II several investigators allowed their patients to assume more normal levels of physical and social activity (17-20). They confirmed that there was no increased risk of reinfarction in patients who, after recovery from an acute episode, had resumed the mode of life similar to that which preceded the initial attack.

* This study was supported in part by Public Health Service Research Grant HE-06304 from the National Heart Institute, Bethesda, Maryland, a grant from the Republic Steel Corporation through the Health Fund of Greater Cleveland, and grants from Mr. and Mrs. William H. Loveman and Mr. and Mrs. Edgar Weil.

Concommitantly, epidemiological studies brought to light the lower mortality and morbidity from coronary disease in subjects with physically demanding occupations (21-24). In the past twenty-five years this observation has led to an enormous increase in our clinical knowledge, a very important part of which has been the identification of those people most likely to develop clinical coronary heart disease and the factors which are associated with this high risk (23, 25-28). In addition more detailed study of patients with acute myocardial infarct has yielded much information relating to modes of sudden death, namely cardiac arrhythmias, and new methods for their control (29-32).

As the result of these advances it has become practical to pose the question, "Can physical conditioning be of therapeutic value in the treatment of coronary heart disease?" and "Can it be of preventive value when applied to subjects who are identified as having an increased risk of heart attack?" If the position is taken that physical activity is a "normal" healthy component of man's existence, and if one of the aims of the health professions is to help restore and maintain health, then the question must be asked "How can one practically help the coronary patient to attain as optimal a state of health as possible (including the restoration or initiation of physical activity)?"

On the basis of our experience in the past eight years we believe that physical conditioning can be of therapeutic value to coronary subjects (atherosclerotic heart disease, ASHD), and it may be of preventive value in normal coronary prone subjects (NCP) (25, 33, 34). Furthermore we are impressed that the general state of inactivity (hypokinetic mode of life) prevalent in our country is in itself an abnormal state (35). ASHD and NCP subjects and normal individuals should engage in regular physical activity commensurate with their abilities and physical limitations in order to maintain a general state of optimal health. For ASHD and NCP subjects it becomes important to determine the extent of potential cardiac limitation, to identify the factors which comprise this limitation, and to devise means by which regular physical activity may be enhanced.

Many people, sometime during their lives, get the urge to become physically active. Frequently this drive is expressed as a one-time or two-time all-out effort to compete with their sons at a sport such as basketball, which may be detrimental. Occasionally the desire is expressed to enter into a training program, but interest wanes rapidly, and patience wears thin, unless physical conditioning can be made attractive. A demand for physical training is infrequently made by a person who is resolute in his intentions to participate sytematically and to achieve and maintain a reasonable constant level of "fitness." Coronary subjects or normal subjects who have become frightened by the prospect of developing coronary disease may consult a physical educator out of anxiety about their health. The number, strength, and type of motives which accompany prospective participants in a training program are many and differ considerably. It is the task of the physical educator to evaluate the individual inquiries, encourage interest, and provide a long range rational approach to satisfying the actual as well as the self-conceived needs of the participants. A large segment of our adult population has been shown to be coronary prone, i.e. to possess early atherosclerotic lesions in the second and third decade (36), and to develop clinical coronary disease prematurely (37). Exercise stress testing of apparently healthy populations has elicited a significant proportion of abnormal ECG responses and has helped to identify subjects with hitherto undetected myocardial ischemia who are most vulnerable to developing clinical ASHD or sudden death (38, 39). The extent of this "silent disease" has not yet been established. At best the apparently healthy NCP individual differs from the ASHD subject in that he may not have a significantly obstructive atherosclerotic abnormality of his coronary arteries. At worst the NCP subject may have more severe obstructive coronary artery atherosclerosis than the ASHD subject, but differs only in that he has not yet manifested his disease clinically with a "heart attack" or angina pectoris. Under these circumstances the NCP subject may have almost as great a risk of dying from the consequences of coronary atherosclerosis as does the patient whose disease has been identified. In addition to use as a screening procedure, exercise testing, for ASHD subjects, gives valuable information on reasonable, safe limits of effort for an individual, and is particularly useful when applied in vocational counselling and physical reconditioning programs.

Physical training is only part of the overall comprehensive regimen for NCP and ASHD subjects. It is equally important to modify other risk factors: i.e. dietary modification, correction of obesity, discontinuance of smoking, adequate medical management of hypertension and diabetes, decreasing emotional tension, as well as enhancing physical activity (exercise, sleep, relaxation), even though experimental confirmation of this necessity may be distant.

The programs to be described here have been conducted on a large scale, as part of the Case Western Reserve University, Jewish Community Feasibility Study (CWRU-JCC),* and on a smaller scale as a pilot study at the Veterans Administration Hospital, Cleveland, Ohio (CVAH).† From these two personal experiences an attempt will be made to offer practical suggestions for the initial evaluation and physical training of subjects with actual and potential coronary heart disease. A second aim of this chapter is to discuss some of the potential benefits and hazards of "fitness" programs, and to offer new information which bears on some of the effects of physical training.

METHODS AND MATERIALS
CWRU - JCC Study

The CWRU-JCC study was conducted from 1961 to 1967. Six hundred and fifty-six nonrandomized males of whom 254 had ASHD participated in the study (Fig. 8-1). The subjects of this intervention study were white, middle-aged, middle and upper class men who were referred to the program by their physicians. They continued to look to their private physicians for their overall medical care. At the onset of the feasibility study, no attempt was made to gather a true random sample or a "control" group. A comparison group consisted of 194 coronary-stricken, age-matched, sex-matched, and color-matched subjects concurrently evaluated in a work classification clinic. They were followed over the same period of time as the intervention subjects.

---

* Principal Investigator: H. K. Hellerstein. Collaborators: I. Bernstein, A. Burlando, C. W. Dupertuis, G. Feil, E. Friedman, A. Goldbarg, E. Z. Hirsch, T. Hornsten, H. Maistelman, S. Marik, F. Plotkin, J. D. Radke, R. Ricklin, S. H. Salzman, and O. Winkler.

† Principal coinvestigators: E. Z. Hirsch and C. A. Macleod. Assisted by: W. Adad, B. Befeler, J. F. Cullinan, A. Gibbons, P. Gould, A. Kamen, and H. Schwartz.

J.C.C. FEASIBILITY STUDY

656 Nonrandomized males
    402 Normal coronary-prone subjects. Average age $=$ 45 yrs.
    254 Coronary heart disease (angina and/or documented M. I.)
            Average age $=$ 48.8 YRS.
            Followed for 697 subject-years (average $=$ 2.7 yrs.)
      0   Congestive heart failure

        Average weight gain since 25 yrs. old $=$ 19 lbs.
        Subjects greater than 15 percent overweight $=$ 28%
        Average fitness level at outset (O_2/Kg BW) $=$ 25 ML.

    Professional $=$ 32%   Businessmen $=$ 20%
    Managerial $=$ 22%   Salesmen $=$ 17%

Cigarette smokers $=$ 47%   Average work week $=$ 50 hrs.

        Type A personality classification $=$ 72%
        MMPI scores generally high in: depression
                                        hypochondriasis
                                        hysteria

Figure 8-1. Some characteristics of the CWRU-JCC study population.

Of the 656 subjects in the intervention program, 402 were categorized as normal coronary-prone subjects (NCP) and 254 as having coronary heart disease (ASHD). Two hundred and three subjects had clinically documented angina pectoris, myocardial infarction, or angina pectoris with myocardial infarction. The remaining fifty-one subjects had "silent coronary artery disease," that is QRS changes consistent with the Minnesota code for myocardial infarction and abnormal exercise electrocardiographic tests with ischemia, but no clinically documented episodes. Of the subjects with manifest coronary disease, 60 percent had angina pectoris. None had congestive heart failure.

The coronary-stricken subjects were followed for a total of 697 subject years, with an average of 2.7 years. At the time of the intake into the study the average age of the NCP subjects was forty-five years and of the ASHD subjects 48.8 years. Since the age of twenty-five years, the body weight had increased on an average of nineteen pounds; 28 percent of the subjects were more than 15 percent over-weight. The overall physical fitness, as determined by computing pre-dicted maximal oxygen uptake, was low compared to Scandinavians of the same age and sex (Fig. 8-2). Thirty-two percent of the

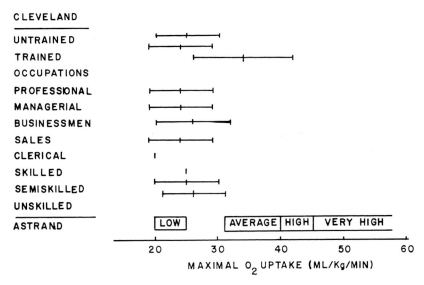

Figure 8-2. Maximal oxygen uptake of study subjects on intake in the con-ditioning program was low compared with Åstrand's Swedish males.

subjects were professionals (physicians, dentists, engineers, phar-macists, lawyers); 22 percent, managerials; 20 percent, businessmen and executives; 17 percent, salesmen; and the remainder, semiskilled workers. Only one percent was unskilled. They worked on an average more than fifty hours a week. Forty-seven percent smoked cigarettes. Seventy-two percent possessed the behavioral characteristics of Type A personality, classified according to the method of Rosenman and Friedman (40, 41). In general, their scores on the depression (D), hyprochondriasis (HS), and hysteria (HY) scales of the Minnesota Personality Inventory (42) were elevated (41).

Indications and contraindications for participation in programs planned to enhance physical fitness are listed in Table 8-I. As a general rule NCP and ASHD subjects would not be accepted to a physical conditioning program:

1. If the facilities lacked supervision and equipment to cope with demands of the program and complications if they should arise.
2. If a subject's illness precluded the ability to exercise in the program.
3. If a subject's illness might be worsened by a training program (such as uncontrolled congestive heart failure or untreated hypertension).

TABLE 8-I

INDICATIONS AND CONTRAINDICATIONS FOR PARTICIPATION IN PROGRAMS PLANNED TO ENHANCE PHYSICAL FITNESS

	Contraindications	
Indications	*Cardiovascular*	*Others*
Normal Subjects, especially highly coronary prone, general deconditioning, neurocirculatory asthenia, before and after surgery*	Severe (80-90%) stenosis of three major coronary arteries	Uncontrolled diabetes mellitus
	Rapidly progressing angina	Marked obesity
	Impending infarction	Deforming arthritis*
	Massive ventricular aneurysm	Skeletal-muscle disorders
Arteriosclerotic Heart Disease*	Congestive failure	Psychosis
Intermittent Claudication*	Arrhythmias:	Recent pulmonary embolism
Pulmonary Disease*	ventricular tachycardia	Severe varicose veins with thrombophlebitis, phlebothrombosis
	2nd, 3rd A-V block	
	fixed ventricular rate pacemaker	Anemia
	untreated artrial fibrillation	Central nervous system disease*
	ventricular premature beats at rest which increase with exercise	CAUTION: SUBJECTS WHO ARE RECEIVING DRUGS: reserpine, propranolol, guanethidine, ganglionic blockers, procaine amide, quinidine
	Valvular disease moderate to severe	
	Outflow obstruction	
	Uncontrolled hypertension	

* Selected cases.

These guidelines were followed in the study. Subjects were accepted only after:

1. They, *and their wives,* had been given a detailed account of the entire program, including the research objectives and methods of study, the extent of their commitment, and a discussion of potential risks and the possible benefits.
2. At least one and preferably more weeks interim period had transpired during which the subjects were instructed to consult

their private physicians for advice and to contact the program directors for further information, if needed.

3. The subjects submitted a written request for participation, a signed referral, and a resume of a recent medical examination by their private physicians.

Medical History

Medical cardiovascular records included a detailed personal history of coronary disease in the subjects and in their families. Subjects were specifically questioned about the presence of previously documented myocardial infarcts, angina pectoris, dyspnea either at rest or with exertion, ankle edema, and other signs of congestive heart failure. They were questioned about the presence of diabetes mellitus, gout, peptic ulcer, and hypertension. A detailed history of cigarette smoking and other usage of tobacco was obtained.

Physical Examination

Cardiovascular physical examination included examination of the ocular fundi, chest, heart, and condition of arterial pulses. At the beginning of the examination right and left arm blood pressures were measured by the cuff method with the subjects in the sitting position. Repeat measurements were made in the left arm after ten and fifteen minutes. Perception of somatic pain was estimated by response to pressure over the styloid process (Libman's sign). Height and weight were measured, and the size of the body frame was estimated by measurements of the depth of the chest, the width of the shoulder, chest, and hips, and the girth of the ankles. The amount of subcutaneous fat was estimated by caliper measurements of vertical fat folds of chest, abdomen, iliac crest, posterior thigh, and triceps. Somatotype was determined from photographs according to the method of Sheldon and Dupertuis (43). The percentage overweight was computed according to tables established by the Metropolitan Life Insurance Company.

Evaluation of Coronary Proneness

The extent of coronary proneness of each individual was assessed on the basis of the number of his coronary risk factors. These included documented past history and family history of coronary disease, present history of angina pectoris and/or signs of congestive heart failure, hypertension, high fat diet, cigarette smoking, obesity, degree of endomesomorphy, personal or family history of heart disease, diabetes mellitus, peptic ulcer or gout, unexplained abnormality of vital capacity, nonspecific changes in the resting ECG, ischemic ST-T changes in the exercise ECG, and serum cholesterol (greater than 250 mg/100 ml).

Laboratory Studies

Total and one second vital capacity were measured on a Collin's Vitalometer. A supine resting standard 12 lead ECG was recorded. The ECG response to Flack test (Valsalva maneuver) was recorded.

Determination of Physical Fitness

Physical fitness was assessed with a modified von Dobëln bicycle (44, 45). A blood pressure cuff attached to a mercury sphygmomanometer was placed on the upper left arm. The subjects sat on a bicycle for at least three minutes. After this, three blood pressure readings were recorded in rapid succession. The subjects then underwent a forty-five-second period of hyperventilation during which the ECG was recorded. Each subject then pedalled for a period of six minutes with intervening rest periods of four minutes each, beginning at a level of 150 kilopond meters per minute (KPM/min)* and increasing in increments of 150 KPM/min until a heart rate of 150 beats per minute was reached. A subject who was considered relatively physically fit initially underwent a warm-up period pedalling against zero resistence for at least four minutes after which he began exercise at either 450 to 600 KPM. ECGs were recorded at intervals of one minute during work and rest. Blood pressure was measured in the left arm during the first and fifth minute of work and during the third minute of rest.

Physical fitness was characterized by responses of the heart rate and blood pressure. The work load producing a heart rate of 150

---

* One kilopond is the force exerted when a mass of one kilogram is subjected to the normal force of gravity.

beats per minute, Work Load 150 (WL_{150}), and predicted maximal oxygen uptake per kilogram of body weight were calculated according to the methods of Åstrand (46) and Lange-Andersen (47). WL_{150} per kilogram of body weight was calculated. A minimal heart rate of 135 beats per minute was used to extrapolate to WL_{150}. An indirect measure of myocardial oxygen consumption (48, 49) was obtained from the product of heart rate and systolic blood pressure (HR $\times$ SBP), which was computed for the last minute of exercise at each work level and expressed in units times 10^2.

The exercise ECGs were analyzed according to the methods of Lester *et al.*, i.e. in terms of ST-T displacement and the slope of the first 0.08 seconds of the ST segment (50). Electrodes for ECG monitoring were arranged according to a modified system of Arbaquez *et al.* (51). Unipolar and bipolar ECG leads were recorded. Each lead for every work load was categorized as being normal, borderline, or abnormal (52). The ECGs of follow-up tests were evaluated in the same manner, and comparisons between tests were made for the same lead at identical external work loads. Improvement or deterioration of the exercise ECG was judged as a change of ECG category.

Psychological Evaluation

Psychological evaluations included a structured interview by a trained staff member, the Holzmann ink blot test,* and the Minnesota Multiphasic Personality Index (MMPI) (42). Special attention was paid to the level of scores on the Hysteria (H) and Hypochondriasis (HS) scales. ASHD subjects were found to have a high degree of depression as judged by MMPI profile. Our subjects had an average profile similar to those of class IIB and IIC subjects with ASHD studied in the Cleveland Work Classification Clinic between 1950 and 1963 (53). Subjects with more serious ASHD had higher depression scores. Angina pectoris and myocardial infarction were associated with even higher depression scores. This relation also held true for the psychasthenia (Pt) scale.

---

* E. Friedman's modification of Holtzman ink blot technique. Available from Psychological Corp., 304 E. 45th St., New York, N.Y. 10017.

Training Categories

Exercise prescription was made on the basis of the above determinations. Subjects were classified into general groups on the basis of type and extent of abnormalities:

Trained 1 (T1)—No limitations in a trained male.

Trained 2 (T2)—10%-20% overweight.

Untrained 1 (U1)—Same as T1 except untrained response to exercise.

Untrained 2 (U2)—Same as T2 except untrained.

Limited 1 (L1)—Significant family history or generally correctable abnormalities, normal "untrained" in response to exercise test.

Limited 2 (L2)—Normal "untrained" response to exercise test plus more severe noncardiac abnormalities or other evidence of possible cardiac disease.

Supervised 1 (S1)—Symptoms or signs of coronary disease or hypertensive cardiovascular disease.

Supervised 2 (S2)—Evidence of severe coronary disease.

For detailed enumeration of criteria for classification see Appendix I.

Subjects in each group had a different target for training and underwent training at individualized intensities and rates of progress dependent upon their response to our standard exercise test. Subjects were required to attend one-hour sessions three times a week. Each session included thirty minutes of calisthenics, ten to fifteen minutes of run-walk sequences, and fifteen minutes of recreational activity. Subjects in the trained group (T1) started calisthenics at two thirds of the allotted counts for each calisthenic exercise. In subsequent sessions they increased the percentage as rapidly as they acclimated to the activity. Likewise they gradually increased the duration and speed of run-walk sequences. Figure 8-3 outlines the prescription. Calisthenic routines were standardized (see Discussion).

In the untrained, limited, and supervised groups progressively greater restrictions were placed on their exercise regimens, and they trained at slower rates (Fig. 8-4, 8-5, and 8-6). This frequently meant that, in the beginning, subjects were training at paces which were *less demanding* than those which they themselves might choose. Dur-

T 1 - T 2

WEEK	1	2	3	4	5	6	7	8	9	10	11	12
Calisthenics Count												
24	18	18	24	-	-	-	-	-	-	-	-	-
36	27	27	36	-	-	-	-	-	-	-	-	-
48	36	36	48	-	-	-	-	-	-	-	-	-
Restrictions	None			Improve Technique								
TRACK												
RUN	2	3	4	5	6	7	7	8	9	10	11	12
WALK	2	2	2	2	3	3	3	3	3	3	3	3
SEQUENCES..	2	2	2	2	2	2	2	2	2	1	1	1
(T 2)	2	2	3	4	5	6	6	7	8	9	10	12
	2	2	2	2	2	3	3	3	3	3	3	3
	2	2	2	2	2	2	2	2	2	2	1	1

Recreation
Restrictions: None

Figure 8-3. General exercise prescription for groups T₁ and T₂. The numbers in "Calisthenics" refer to the number of times each exercise is performed. Those in "Track, Run, Walk" refer to laps approximately 20 laps per mile). "Sequences" denotes the number of times the "Run-walk" patterns are executed in a training session.

ing the initial period it was incumbent upon the program designer to prevent dropout. This was best done with "recreational activities," by devising interesting activities and by encouraging the subjects frequently.

Physical Training

The essential ingredient in a physical training program for NCP and ASHD subjects is frequent communication and feedback between the subjects and supervisors. In the CWRU-JCC study this was established through the use of written records for which the subjects were responsible. Appendix II shows a reproduction of the forms used. The activities listed in the "recreational activity" section and referred to, by designated letter symbol, in Fig. 8-6 are those which were *not* restricted in the S1 and S2 groups. Exercise prescriptions were written on this form and attendance recorded by the participant. The record was returned to the physical educator monthly and a new prescription was issued. Criteria for

U 1 - U 2

WEEK	1	2	3	4	5	6	7	8	9	10	11	12
Calisthenics Count												
24	12	18	18	24	-	-	-	-	-	-	-	-
36	18	27	27	36	-	-	-	-	-	-	-	-
48	24	36	36	48	-	-	-	-	-	-	-	-
(U 2)	12	18	18	24	-	-	-	-	-	-	-	-
	18	27	27	36	-	-	-	-	-	-	-	-
	24	36	36	48	-	-	-	-	-	-	-	-
Restrictions	None											
TRACK												
RUN	1	2	2	3	4	5	5	6	7	8	9	10
WALK	1	2	2	2	2	2	2	3	3	3	3	3
SEQUENCES..	3	2	2	2	2	2	2	2	2	2	2	1
(U 2)	½	1	1	2	3	4	4	5	6	7	8	9
	1	1	1	2	2	2	2	2	3	3	3	3
	3	3	3	2	2	2	2	2	2	2	2	2

Recreation Restrictions: None

Figure 8-4. General exercise prescription for groups U_1 and U_2.

L 1 - L 2

WEEK	1	2	3	4	5	6	7	8	9	10	11	12
Calisthenics Count												
24	12	12	15	18	18	24	-	-	-	-	-	-
36	18	18	21	27	27	36	-	-	-	-	-	-
48	24	24	27	36	36	48	-	-	-	-	-	-
Restrictions	None											
TRACK												
RUN	½	1	1	1	2	3	3	4	5	6	7	7
WALK	1	1	1	1	2	2	2	2	2	3	3	3
SEQUENCES...	3	3	4	5	2	2	2	2	2	2	3	3
(L 2)	½	1	1	1	1	2	2	3	4	5	6	6
	1	1	1	1	1	2	2	2	2	2	3	3
	3	2	3	4	5	2	2	2	2	2	3	3

Recreation Restrictions: No Competition - May compete with our approval
Other activities O.K.

Figure 8-5. General exercise prescription for groups L_1 and L_2.

S 1 - S 2

WEEK	1	2	3	4	5	6	7	8	9	10	11	12
Calisthenics Count												
24	12	12	12	12	18	18	18	24	24	24	24	24
36	18	18	21	21	27	27	27	36	36	36	36	36
48	24	24	27	27	36	36	36	48	48	48	48	48
(S 2)	12	12	12	12	18	18	18	24	24	24	24	
	18	18	21	21	27	27	27	36	36	36	36	
	24	24	27	27	36	36	36	48	48	48	48	

Restrictions S 1: No Floor Exercise
No Hops - First Month
Beginning with Week Five - ½ Count on Hops

Restrictions S 2: No Floor Exercise
No Hops

TRACK	1	2	3	4	5	6	7	8	9	10	11	12
RUN	½	½	½	1	1	1	1	1	2	3	4	5
WALK	1	1	1	2	2	2	2	2	3	3	3	3
SEQUENCES...	3	3	3	3	3	4	4	5	2	2	2	2
					½	½	1	1	1	2	2	
(S 2)	10 Min.	10 Min.	20 Min.	20 Min.	3	3	1	1	1	2	2	
					2	2	3	2	3	3	2	

Recreation Restrictions: (S 1)   May Do A, B, C, D, E (w/1 plate), J.K.
No competition

(S 2)   May Do B, D, E (w1 plate), J.K.
No competition

Figure 8-6. General exercise prescription for groups S₁ and S₂. The letter designations in "Recreation restrictions" are defined in "Monthly Exercise Prescription" (Appendix II).

advancement in the program was related to improvement and to adherence (Fig. 8-7). A home exercise plan was incorporated for some participants consisting of calisthenics slightly less demanding than those conducted in the calisthenics classes. All subjects attended the same classes even though each individual followed his specific prescription. Subjects in the S1 and S2 groups were not monitored during physical training.

The exercise prescription for groups S1 and S2 (Fig. 8-6) were generally conservative at the outset. The subjects were instructed to take nitroglycerin prophylatically and frequently, and to rest for two to five minutes when symptoms appeared before resuming

CRITERIA FOR ADVANCEMENT IN THE
TRAINING PROGRAM

Attendance	*Program*
1. 12 Sessions or more per month	Advancement to next month's activity program
2. 10-11 sessions per month	Repeat previous week's program
3. 8-9 Sessions per month	Repeat two week's program
4. 6-7 Sessions per month	Repeat three week's program
5. 5 or less sessions per month	Repeat entire month's program
6. Home exercise plan 15 minutes / day 7 days / week	Increases attendance record by two sessions

7. *Any unusual symptoms are to be reported to the staff immediately*

Figure 8-7. Criteria are used as guidelines for safety, not as rigid rules.

activity. Supervision by a physical educator was maintained. The concept of gradual increase in activity was stressed.

During the course of physical training, when it became apparent that optimal fitness had been attained, in accordance with cardiac limitations and appropriate drug therapy, a level of exercise slightly below that which had been attained was prescribed as a regular routine for the future. By this time the subject had become proficient in the use of exercise principles, and supervision was relaxed. Exercise reports and prescriptions continued. Rules for advancement enumerated in Fig. 8-7 continued to apply, if the subjects were not able to exercise for reasons other than their coronary disease. In cases where a high level of fitness had been achieved, and a period of bed rest or cardiac disability had supervened, the subjects assumed training at a low level and advanced as tolerated (see Discussion). Incorporated into future exercise prescriptions was the provision for long walks with distance goals. When the pattern of run-walk activity had reached maximum for a given subject, he was given a goal such as one mile a day to be accomplished in a manner arrived at during training (provided that the subject's symptoms had not changed).

CVAH PILOT STUDY

Histories, physical examination, chest x-rays, and resting 12 lead ECGs were obtained. Exercise tests were conducted in a similar manner to CWRU-JCC study. ECG monitoring was accomplished with the use of a bipolar lead system with the reference electrode on the forehead and the exploring electrodes at the $V_{1.5}$, V_4, and V_6 chest positions (54, 55). The "lead 1" position on an ECG recorder was used. Complexes obtained with these three leads approximated V_2, V_4, and V_6 of the resting 12 lead ECG. The usual German silver electrodes were applied with the aid of rubber straps. To minimize interference from body motion a thin strip of gauze saturated with conducting jelly was placed between the electrode and the skin. The work load was determined at which definitely abnormal ECG responses occurred. Nitroglycerin was subsequently given sublingually. The previous work load was repeated, and the test continued at higher stress until recurrence of abnormalities. Two subjects with severe angina pectoris underwent a number of exercise tests, without medication, and after several days of medication (oral and sublingual isosorbide dinitrate, propranolol, digoxin, and a combination of the drugs). These two subjects continued to take isosorbide dinitrate and propranolol orally during the training period to assess these drugs as adjuncts to physical training. At intervals in the program these drugs were discontinued selectively, and exercise tests were repeated. Following the study a series of exercise tests were performed on these two subjects with double blind administration of drugs (and placebo).

Cardiac catheterization was carried out before and six to nine months after physical training while subjects were in a steady state of fitness. Coronary cineangiograms and additional cardiac function studies were performed on seven subjects. The complete protocol included four observational periods prior to obtaining cineangiograms: rest, isoproterenol infusion, recovery (30 min after the end of isoproterenol infusion), and exercise. The following parameters were recorded during these periods: arterial and left ventricular pressures, cardiac output, arterial and coronary sinus blood samples for lactic acid, oxygen saturation, and in some cases serum enzyme and potassium levels. Following this, selective coronary cineangiograms and ventriculograms were obtained. The same dose-rate infusion of isoproterenol and the same level of exercise were employed before and after training. Cineangiograms were made with a six-inch image intensifier, using a 35-mm camera at sixty frames per second, and a fine grain cine developer. All films viewed by several independent observers were judged to be of uniformly excellent quality.

Cholesterol turnover studies according to the method of Goodman and Noble (56) were performed on eleven subjects before and after physical training. Eight subjects trained, and three remained as untrained controls. Ten subjects had ASHD. The remaining subject had hypercholesterolemia (Fredrickson's type II classification) (57). Serum cholesterol and triglyceride levels were determined on weekly blood samples throughout the pretraining, training, and posttraining periods. Triglyceride turnover studies were carried out as well. Intravenous glucose tolerance was determined before and after physical training.

Detailed results of these pilot studies will be reported elsewhere. Some of the data are included here, inasmuch as they have helped to substantially modify our approach to physical training of the ASHD subject.

In the CVAH pilot study exercise prescriptions were not given initially. Instead monitored bicycle ergometer training exercises were performed for the first two to four weeks of training. Gradually the bicycle activity was reduced as jogging and swimming were increased. Calisthenics were not used. In asymptomatic subjects with normal ECG and blood pressure responses to the initial training regimen monitoring was discontinued after several sessions. Abnormal responders were taught how to apply and care for their electrodes and recorded their training activities and symptomatic responses in specific detail (Fig. 8-8). Exercise included a warm-up period, followed by sequences of 0.5 to 1 minute ascending work loads with intervening periods of "free wheeling" against zero resistance. Lighter work loads of longer duration (2 to 4 min) were interspersed and increased as training advanced. At the beginning of every exercise session each participant carried out a sequence of two-minute exercise periods at zero resistance, 150 KPM/min, 300 KPM/min, etc., until symptoms

NOTATION OF PAIN

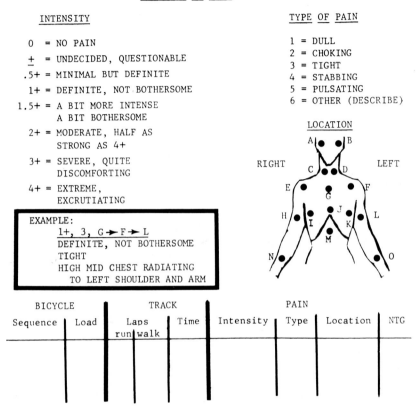

INTENSITY

0 = NO PAIN

± = UNDECIDED, QUESTIONABLE

.5+ = MINIMAL BUT DEFINITE

1+ = DEFINITE, NOT BOTHERSOME

1.5+ = A BIT MORE INTENSE
       A BIT BOTHERSOME

2+ = MODERATE, HALF AS
     STRONG AS 4+

3+ = SEVERE, QUITE
     DISCOMFORTING

4+ = EXTREME,
     EXCRUTIATING

TYPE OF PAIN

1 = DULL
2 = CHOKING
3 = TIGHT
4 = STABBING
5 = PULSATING
6 = OTHER (DESCRIBE)

LOCATION

RIGHT   LEFT

EXAMPLE:
    1+, 3, G ➤ F ➤ L
DEFINITE, NOT BOTHERSOME
TIGHT
HIGH MID CHEST RADIATING
    TO LEFT SHOULDER AND ARM

| BICYCLE | | TRACK | | PAIN | | | |
Sequence	Load	Laps run|walk	Time	Intensity	Type	Location	NTG

Figure 8-8. Guide and form used by subjects to describe their exercise during training sessions. Subjects were able to utilize this coding method and record in detail their symptoms.

and ECG changes appeared. This sequence served as a comparative effort test from session to session. Following this, sublingual nitroglycerin was administered, and further exercise was performed. Nitroglycerin was taken every five to 10 minutes until headache ensued, regardless of whether or not the subjects experienced angina. In addition to symptoms each participant recorded the times at which nitroglycerin, 0.3 mg, was used (Fig. 8-8). After two to eight weeks, cycling was interspersed with run-walk sequences on a track. Here the subjects were monitored at the end of each track sequence, by

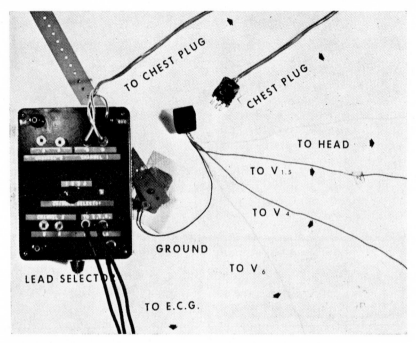

Figure 8-9. Simple three channel switchbox used for ECG monitoring of multiple simultaneous exercise procedures is interposed between electrodes and an ordinary ECG recorder. A plug situated on the subjects chest, contributes to the mobility of the unit. Subjects learn to apply and care for their own electrodes. The right arm ECG lead is attached to the head electrode. The left arm ECG lead is used as the exploring electrode, which is positioned through the lead selector switch.

plugging their chest electrodes into a lead wire which connected them to a switch box and the ECG recorder. Figure 8-9 shows the switch box which was used at the CVAH. It was designed to monitor sequentially three subjects performing simultaneously on the bicycle or up to eight subjects following running. It is capable of switching to one of three input channels, and to one of three bipolar or unipolar leads.

Details of the equipment have been included to emphasize that the adequate monitoring of several subjects at a time can be achieved with a readily available, single-channel ECG recorder and a low-cost lead switch box. The practicality of this method increases with the number of subjects being monitored. In contrast, monitoring several subjects at a time by ECG telemetry and/or oscillographic display is costly and much more complex, notwithstanding other potential benefits of such equipment.

In the CVAH study all of the so-called asymptomatic ASHD subjects who responded abnormally to the effort test exhibited at least slight chest discomfort at strenuous work loads. These symptoms were reproducible on repeated tests and generally correlated well with the appearance and recession of ECG abnormalities. This indicated to the subjects that their cardiac limitation had been reached. Breathlessness appeared frequently in conjunction with chest pain and in some subjects became the predominant symptom as chest pain improved during training. Its disappearance following exercise paralleled that of chest pain. Pulmonary edema or other manifestations of congestive heart failure did not appear in any subject. (Although very high values for left ventricular end-diastolic pressures were recorded during exercise in some subjects before training, they remained subsequently unchanged.) One of us (E. Z. H.) monitored the abnormal responders and, on the basis of performance of the previous effort, instructed the subjects on the next task. In many instances after a number of monitoring sessions, when the reproducibility of ECG abnormalities and the pattern of chest pain occurrence in relation to these abnormalities were established, subjects were allowed to continue training unmonitored, but with electrodes in place. They repeated familiar sequences using chest pain as the limiting guideline. The subjects uniformly became expert in detecting slight chest sensations premonitory to subsequent pain and in predicting the time of onset and progression of severity of the pain once it became established. *The onset of chest pain was not an indication to stop.* Progression of the pain to 2+ was used instead (Fig. 8-8). In most instances both pain and ECG abnormalities subsided within fifteen to thirty seconds of recovery. In only two of more than five thousand pain episodes did the abnormalities last for more than two minutes following exercise. In one of the two instances of prolonged chest pain (5 min) the subject had elected to run extra laps not in keeping with anticipated progress in the program. The other instance was unexpected in a subject who had a long history of easily anticipatable exercise chest pain. Serum enzyme studies on both of these subjects revealed no elevations. Their subsequent clinical state was unchanged.

Modification of the Bicycle Exercise Test

In order to facilitate exercise testing, we have tried a modification of the above mentioned bicycle test at the CVAH. The duration of exercise has been reduced from six to three minutes with intervening rest periods of two minutes each. This modification decreases the total time required for the test, although it sacrifices the steady state. However, the heart rates are reproducible and comparable to those obtained with longer exercise periods. The feature of intermittent rest between increments of effort during the exercise test has been retained specifically. Since effort induced ECG change and arrhythmias often appear in the immediate post-exercise period, they should be identified before the subject exercises at a high work load. In the absence of intervening rest periods, these abnormalities may appear *during* subsequent higher work loads and be more serious and difficult to manage.

The arm cuff blood pressure is obtained in a control period and during the third minute of exercise, with the unclenched hand raised from the handle bar. Five-second strips of ECG are recorded before exercise, at the first and second minute of each work load, and at each minute of recovery. A continuous record is obtained during the last ten seconds of each work load and the first thirty seconds of recovery. After completion of the thirty-second recovery ECG from the highest work load, the subject tapers off by pedalling against zero resistence for four minutes then walks briskly to avoid postexercise bradycardia and hypotension.

Since the CWRU-JCC study was completed it has become the accepted practice to use a bipolar lead system, rather than a unipolar system, with the reference electrode in the right upper chest or head and the exploring electrode over the left precordium (54, 55).

RESULTS

CWRU - JCC Study

Adherence and Mortality

The CWRU-JCC study was designed to determine the feasibility of carrying out a multifactoral reconditioning program on NCP and ASHD subjects primarily as regards adherence and mortality. Over a six-year period, adherence to the training sessions averaged approximately 50 percent attendance to 10 to 12 sessions per month and an additional 20 percent for 4 to 9.9 sessions per month.

Fitness and improvement in abnormal ECG responses to exercise occurred in ASHD subjects and those with initially abnormal ECG responses who attended an average of at least two sessions per week (grade 3 in Fig. 8-10). More frequent attendance was not associated

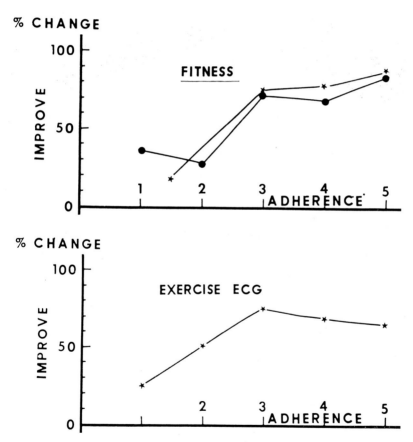

Figure 8-10. Relation of adherence to training program to improvement in physical fitness and in the exercise ECG. The stars indicate subjects with abnormal exercise ECGs on entry into the program. The solid dots represent the total ASHD population. Adherence is graded 1 to 5 (See text).

with linear degrees of improvement. Instead, a plateau was reached in both parameters.

Our experience also indicates that untrained NCP and ASHD subjects frequently have higher systolic blood pressure responses to standard effort before physical training than after fitness has been achieved. This constitutes the entity called "exertional hypertension" and suggests that the myocardial oxygen demand is greater than that which is imposed by the same work load on a trained subject.

At the termination of the CWRU-JCC study, there had been 12 deaths in 254 ASHD subjects with 697 subject years experience. Eleven of these deaths were due to ASHD. The ASHD mortality was therefore 1.6 deaths per hundred subject years. During the following year and one-half of follow-up five more deaths occurred. Over one thousand patient years had accumulated, and the ASHD mortality remained at 1.7 deaths per hundred subject years. When the study terminated, medical records were retrieved from the Cleveland Work Classification Clinic, and 194 subjects were matched with the study subjects for age, diagnosis, functional and therapeutic classification (according to the American Heart Association), and approximate date of initial examination. This group was found to have a mortality of 3.5 deaths per hundred subjects years. In other studies the death rate has been reported to be higher, six deaths per hundred subject years in the natural course of the disease (58).

In the NCP group 10 deaths occurred in 402 subjects during the study and the following year and one-half (1688 total subject years). Seven of these were due to ASHD. The overall mortality was 5.9 per thousand subject years, and the ASHD mortality was 4.2 per thousand subject years.

Recent studies have indicated a high correlation exists between mortality and severity of coronary proneness, ranging from four per thousand subject years in the least coronary prone to twenty per thousand subject years in the more coronary prone groups (59). At present we do not attempt to attribute statistical significance to our results because in the feasibility study no attempt was made to randomize the subjects; however, we can say with reasonable certainty that the mortality rate of physically conditioned ASHD subjects is not greater than subjects who do not undertake a conditioning program.

Two ASHD subjects and two NCP subjects died within several hours of exercising. The only comparison available for these data are studies related to submaximal and maximal effort tests, where sudden death and myocardial infarction have been very rare (60). This finding is corroborated by that of Weinberg *et al.* (61), who found in 428 fatal heart attacks that the greatest number occurred during ordinary mild activity, not during moderate or marked activity. Comparisons such as these are not satisfactory. Instead there is an urgent necessity for a long term study of physical training in ASHD and NCP subjects with suitable controls.

CVAH Pilot Study

Mortality and Morbidity

At CVAH there were neither deaths nor myocardial infarcts during the year of study. Three subjects sustained myocardial infarctions following the completion of the study.

Case 1, G. H., who sustained a myocardial infarct while awaiting admission into the study, sustained the second one several weeks after the study ended. Both infarcts were uncomplicated. During training the subject was held to a minimum regimen because of slight cardiomegaly. The highest level of regular activity obtained was a one-mile run three times a week in modules of 0.05 to 0.1 of a mile (1-2 laps) with intervening rest periods of one to two minutes. Work tolerance improved slightly. The second myocardial infarct was heralded by chest pain at rest starting two days after the previous exercise period. Exercise was discontinued. Chest pain persisted for five days during which his private physician was consulted frequently. The patient was admitted to the CVAH on the sixth day. Changes in the serum enzymes and ECG appeared one day later. Subsequently the subject recovered and two months later resumed his physical activity by slowly retraining. There has been no clinical change during the past year of resumed physical activity comparable to his initial training regimen.

Case 2, M. D., sustained a myocardial infarct four months after detraining. He was an asymptomatic, nonsmoking subject of desired weight with low normal serum cholesterol. His only coronary prone characteristics were a driving restless hyperactive personality and an extremely severe family history. Physical examination and resting 12 lead ECG were normal. The myocardial infarct was heralded by persistent mild chest pain over a period of twenty-four hours without other symptoms. Serum enzyme rose slightly above normal limits, and transient ST-T abnormalities were detected. Recovery was uncomplicated. Coronary angiograms had not been performed previously. At this time they showed complete obstruction of the lateral circumflex artery, 75 percent narrowing of the left anterior descending branch, and severe stenosis ($> 50\%$) in the posterior descending branch of the right coronary artery with abundant intercoronary anastomoses. At no time during training had this subject shown any ECG or other abnormal responses to effort. He had attained three miles per session, running rapidly with an average heart rate of 150. WL_{150} showed 40 percent improvement, from 670 KPM/min to 945 KPM/min.

Case 3, G. K., died from myocardial infarction two months following detraining. He had angiographic evidence of severe narrowing of the left anterior descending artery prior to training. During physical training his WL_{150} improved from 675 KPM/min to 750 KPM/min. Initial abnormal ECG response to exercise disappeared early in training. Adherence was somewhat less than the other subjects. Posttraining angiograms were identical with pretraining films. The subject discontinued exercise following the termination of the study. Sudden chest pain two months later led to a rapid demise. Postmortem examination confirmed the presence of stenosis of the left anterior descending coronary artery exactly as seen on angiography. No evidence of old fibrosis or infarct was seen macroscopically or microscopically in any area of the myocardium. However, a fresh thrombus was identified at the site of the stenosis with changes of early infarction throughout the free wall of the left ventricle. This case was interpreted to indicate that physical activity did not cause myocardial cell death in spite of severe coronary narrowing.

Schettler has reported an increased incidence of deaths in athletes immediately after detraining (62). Cases 2 and 3 fall into this category. It is possible that Shettler's observations may constitute a specific clinical entity. Certainly his report and our small experience suggest that follow-up of trained subjects is important and that subjects be advised against intentional rapid detraining following the regular performance of strenuous exercise. More research into the biological effects of detraining is urgently needed.

Exercise and Myocardial Ischemia

Chest pain and ECG abnormalities are observed commonly in many ASHD subjects undergoing physical training. In order to determine whether these episodes of exercise-induced myocardial ischemia reflect the destructive loss of myocardial tissue in the absence of frank clinical infarction, coronary sinus and arterial enzymes* and potas-

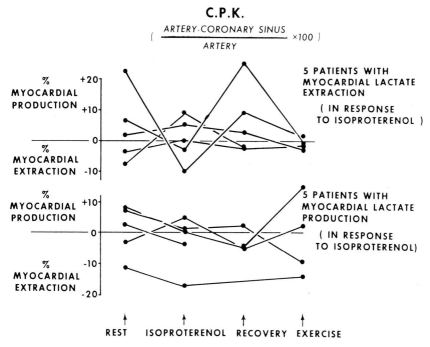

Figure 8-11. Coronary sinus-arterial differences in creatine phosphokinase during four periods at cardiac catheterization related to the behavior of myocardial lactates. Myocardial lactate production is currently thought to reflect anaerobic metabolism, and consequently, to indicate indirectly the presence of myocardial ischemia.

---

* These determinations were performed on previously aliquoted duplicate serum samples, in coded random sequence prior to lactate determination. They were performed by Dr. Charles E. Jackson, Director of the Caylor-Nickel Research Foundation, Bluffton, Indiana. Lactates were likewise determined in duplicate.

Exercise and the Heart

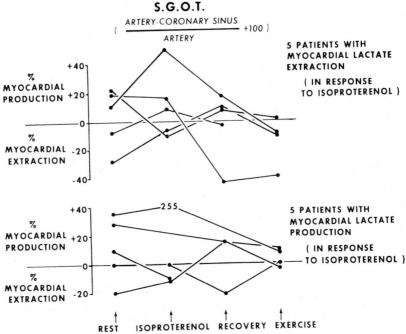

S.G.O.T.

Figure 8-12. Coronary sinus-arterial differences in S. G. O. T. during four periods at cardiac catheterization related to the behavior of myocardial lactates.

sium were studied in ten ASHD subjects. Five subjects showed myocardial lactate production, and five showed normal myocardial lactate extraction during intravenous isoproterenol infusion. There were no differences in serum enzyme levels of these two groups at rest, during isoproterenol infusion, and during moderately severe exercise. Figures 8-11 and 8-12 show no correlation between the arterial-coronary sinus difference of these enzymes and myocardial lactate production.

Potassium concentration in the coronary sinus has been shown to increase during coronary artery ligation in dogs (63). Figure 8-13 shows that the arterial coronary sinus differences in potassium were not related to myocardial lactate production.

These pilot studies suggest that myocardial ischemia, as determined by myocardial lactate production (as well as ECG abnormalities and symptoms which occurred in most instances) under condi-

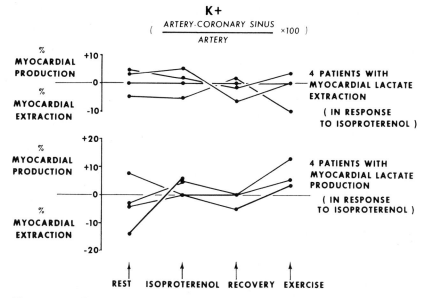

K+

$$\left(\frac{ARTERY\text{-}CORONARY\ SINUS}{ARTERY} \times 100 \right)$$

Figure 8-13. Coronary sinus-arterial differences in potassium during four periods at cardiac catheterization related to the behavior of myocardial lactates.

tions of isoproterenol and effort stresses, probably does not lead to acute undetected myocardial damage in subjects with ASHD. This suggestion is borne out by the absence of clinical deterioration or deterioration of myocardial function on catheterization in subjects before and after physical training (7, 13, 16). In particular no subject in our laboratory has developed congestive heart failure during the nine to twelve months of supervised physical activity.

Cardiac Response to Physical Training

Coronary Arteries. In another subsample of 7 subjects, a detailed study was made of the coronary arterial circulation. Improvements in work tolerance were not associated with gross changes in the anatomy of the coronary arterial system as characterized by coronary arteriograms. The subjects physically trained for six to nine months. They showed no visible change in preexisting coronary arterial lesions. In all subjects, at least one main artery was narrowed by 60 percent or more. Two subjects had major stenoses (exceeding 50%) in two main coronary arteries, and two subjects had major stenoses in all three main vessels. Two subjects had complete occlusion of at least one main vessel, and two others had narrowing of 90 percent or more.

Intercoronary anastomoses were visualized in three subjects, and no intercoronary anastomoses were visualized in four subjects prior to physical training. After six to nine months of training no changes were observed in visualized inter-coronary anastomoses.

In his classic experiment Eckstein (1) showed that physical training enhanced coronary collateral *flow in dogs* with experimentally produced coronary artery stenosis. Coronary angiograms do not measure blood flow, and it is possible that the present technique of coronary arteriography is not sufficiently sensitive to detect small collateral vessels. There are major limitations in extrapolating Eckstein's results to man in that significant anatomical differences exist between the coronary circulations of dog and man. The effect of physical training on blood delivery to the myocardium is not known.

MYOCARDIAL FUNCTION. Changes in myocardial function have been reported following physical training in ASHD subjects. Varnauskas (7) showed a reduction in effective left ventricular work in six ASHD patients. Frick (13) demonstrated a reduction in exercise tension-time index following physical training with no significant change in effective left ventricular work. (Tension-time index reflects myocardial oxygen consumption.) Clausen (16) likewise demonstrated a reduction in tension-time index following physical training in seven patients. We have previously reported comparable effects, i.e. the product of the systolic blood pressure and heart rate during exercise is significantly reduced by training (2, 8, 34, 43, 46, 53).

At the CVAH, of the seven study subjects mentioned above, five improved their work tolerance. (Fig. 8-14). Two subjects with severe angina pectoris underwent training without improvement. Prior to physical training myocardial lactate production during isoproterenol infusion occurred in four of six subjects tested. These results were reflected in arterial lactate responses to effort (Fig. 8-15). All but the two subjects with severe angina showed reduced arterial lactate response following training. Of the subjects with improved WL_{150}, two who initially showed myocardial lactate production continued to show it after physical training. One subject, in whom no pretraining level was obtained, showed myocardial lactate production following train-

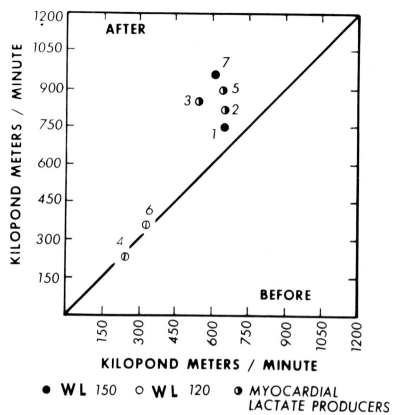

Figure 8-14. Work performance (WL) before and after physical training. Except for two subjects with severe angina (Subjects #4 and #6), WL 150 increased with training without relation to myocardial lactate production.

ing. Two subjects who showed myocardial lactate extraction initially continued to extract lactate following training (Fig. 8-16). Since this study was completed, we have adopted intra-atrial pacing as a more controllable procedure for the study of angina and myocardial lactate production (65, 66).

Thus, despite myocardial lactate production following training, WL_{150} improved considerably (27% to 60%) as did symptoms and ECG response to effort testing in three subjects. The two subjects with severe angina and no improvement in WL_{150} showed no change in myocardial lactate production.

Changes in hemodynamic response to exercise following training

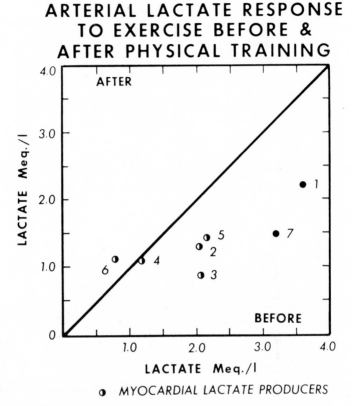

ARTERIAL LACTATE RESPONSE TO EXERCISE BEFORE & AFTER PHYSICAL TRAINING

O MYOCARDIAL LACTATE PRODUCERS

Figure 8-15. Except for two subjects with severe angina (Subjects #4 and #6), arterial lactate levels during standard effort declined without relation to myocardial lactate production.

showed variability which appeared to be related to severity of disease. Severity of disease was defined as a combination of:

1. The number of major coronary vessels affected with stenoses greater than 50 percent.
2. The occurrance of complete obstruction of one or more major coronary vessels.
3. Subjective assessment of left ventricular contractility and ejection fraction at rest by cineangiography.
4. The occurrance of myocardial lactate production during iso-proterenol infusion.

Two subjects were considered minimally affected because of single

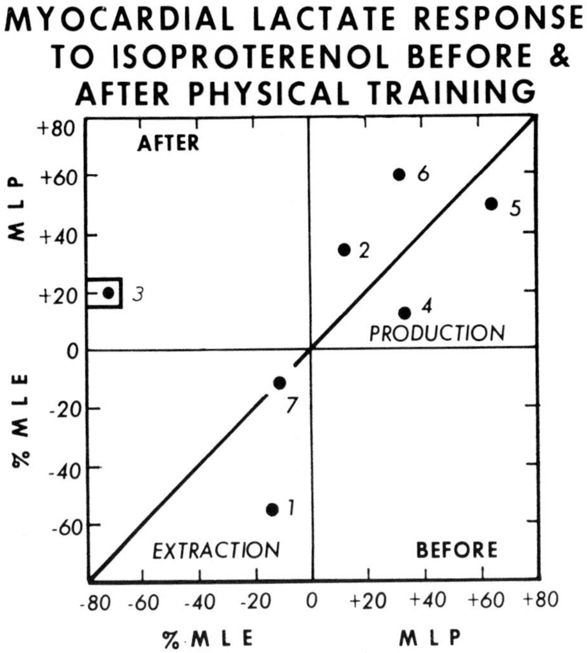

MYOCARDIAL LACTATE RESPONSE TO ISOPROTERENOL BEFORE & AFTER PHYSICAL TRAINING

Figure 8-16. There was no change in the myocardial production or extraction of lactate following physical training. Subject #4, with severe angina, showed myocardial lactate production at rest and during exercise as well. Myocardial lactate production was determined after physical training only, in Subject #3.

vessel stenoses, initial myocardial lactate extraction, and normal resting left ventricular contractility and ejection fraction. These showed no change following training. In response to standard exercise following training WL_{150} improved significantly, with a decrease in heart rate and cardiac index. Stroke index remained unchanged. Left ventricular minute work index and tension-time index decreased. Ejection time index was also reduced, but mean systolic ejection rate was unchanged. In the light of a reduced tension-time index, in addition to reduced left ventricular work, there was no evidence for improved myocardial efficiency. Thus, improved fitness (improved WL_{150}) seemed to result in reduced peripheral demand for blood (decreased cardiac output) and reductions in heart rate and myocardial work; that is, greater "economy" of the oxygen transport system (66) with an adequate cardiac "pump."

At the other extreme are two severely symptomatic subjects who differed in several ways from the two minimally affected subjects in their responses to exercise following physical training. These were the only subjects in the subsample who had complete occlusion of a coronary artery. Initially both showed myocardial lactate production and impaired left ventricular contractility. One showed markedly reduced contractility and reduced ejection fraction both of which improved significantly following training. The other showed less severely impaired contractility, and ejection fraction was within normal limits. Neither changed following training. Following regular stressful physical activity, WL_{150} did not improve in either subject. Heart rate was unchanged and stroke index increased with consequent increase in cardiac index during exercise. In contrast to the previous subjects left ventricular minute work index and mean systolic ejection rate index increased. Tension-time index and ejection time decreased in both groups.

Whole body demands imposed by the standard exercise tests before and after training were identical. The overall response (WL_{150} and exercise ECG) did not change. However the cardiac response seemed to show improvement (increased cardiac index and left ventricular minute work). Increase in stroke index, mean systolic ejection rate index, and a reduction in ejection time index suggested some improvement in myocardial contractility during exercise. Increased left ventricular minute work index in conjunction with reduced tension-time index suggested that the improved cardiac response was accompanied by improved myocardial efficiency. Increases in cardiac index following training are not to be expected in normal sedentary men (66). The left ventricle, then, delivered more blood at an increased velocity per stroke and performed more work with less oxygen consumption in these two subjects.

Three subjects showed features that differed from the other two groups. In common with the minimally affected group, they suffered mild angina or none, and significant improvement in work performance with training took place. They resembled the severely symptomatic group in that all showed myocardial lactate production following training. This group was characterized by coronary artery lesions of a severity intermediate between those of the other two groups. None had complete occlusion of any major vessel, but all had multiple vessel involvement.

The three subjects differed from each other in some of their individual features. In two, following training, the hemodynamic response to exercise resembled that of the minimally affected group, although differing in some respects. Improvement in WL_{150} was associated with reduced left ventricular minute work index and no evidence for improved myocardial efficiency. However, one subject responded in a manner more closely resembling that of the severely symptomatic group. Left ventricular minute work index increased, and tension-time index showed a slight decline suggesting an increase in myocardial efficiency. He differed from the severely symptomatic subjects in that he was able to improve substantially WL_{150} with physical training.

Thus, it is of interest that the two subjects with most severe anatomical and physiological disease showed evidence of greater improvement in myocardial efficiency than those with moderate or minimal disease. Further study with larger numbers of ASHD subjects is required to test adequately the hypotheses suggested above: i.e. that the more severe the mechanical and anatomic abnormalities, the greater the improvement in myocardial function and, that changes in myocardial function may diverge considerably from the overall body response to effort in subjects suitable for training.

Severe Coronary Disease

Observations on two of the subjects with severe anatomic ASHD are reported in order to contrast important differences in their myocardial function, and responses to physical training, and in order to describe our methods for training severely symptomatic subjects.

One subject (Subject #3 in Figs. 8-14, 8-15, and 8-16) was shown by cineangiography to have a 90 percent stenosis in the proximal third of the right coronary artery, 50 percent in the midthird of the left anterior descending coronary artery, 90 percent obstruction more distally, and 50 percent obstruction in the proximal portion of the main marginal branch of the circumflex artery. No intercoronary anastomoses were visualized. The left ventricular contraction appeared to be vigorous. Visually, overall left ventricular volume appeared to be slightly increased, and ejection fraction, slightly reduced. These abnormalities did not change following physical training. This subject demonstrated myocardial lactate production with isoproterenol after training. Left ventricular end-diastolic pressure was normal at rest but significantly elevated during exercise (30 mm Hg). He was asymptomatic. With physical training his WL₁₅₀ increased 50 percent from 550 to 875 KPM/min. Although the subject had had a myocardial infarction, the resting ECG was normal. The initial exercise ECG showed 1 to 2 mm ST-T depression, responsive to nitroglycerin. This abnormality disappeared with training.

This subject trained initially on the bicycle ergometer. He was monitored by ECG for the first four months of training. Although he did not have symptoms he was still given nitroglycerin to tolerance during training sessions. After two and one-half months he began to jog one forty-five-second lap at a time (19.5 laps to the mile) with intervening rest periods. At four and one-half months he was running a mile in twelve minutes. At that time his training sequence was run one lap, walk, and then run, 4, 8, 12, 16, 24 laps with intervening walk periods of two to three minutes each. From that time on he averaged three to five miles per training session, with a decrease in the number and frequency of walk periods. His speed stayed the same. In addition he was taught to swim free style in a relaxed fashion and would swim for ten to twenty minutes at a time. There were no complications arising from this activity. His fitness routine has continued with the addition of volley ball once a week.

The second subject (Subject #4 in Figs. 8-14, 8-15, and 8-16) had an entirely different course. This subject differed initially in that he had not sustained a myocardial infarction, but had experienced angina pectoris for the previous ten years. Cineangiograms revealed complete obstructions near the origin of the right and of the left anterior descending coronary arteries and 70 percent stenosis of the left circumflex artery. Intercoronary anastomoses with heavy retrograde filling were seen. In addition, this subject showed persistent myocardial lactate production at rest and during exercise, as well as during isoproterenol infusion. Left ventricular end-diastolic pressure was elevated at all times at rest and rose to 30 mm Hg during exercise. The cardiac silhouette was borderline in size. Angiographically ventricular volume was within normal limits, but left ventricular contractility was impaired and ejection fraction significantly reduced. Following training contractility and ejection fraction improved significantly. This subject was one of those described above as "severely symptomatic" whose hemodynamic response to exercise showed the most improvement following physical training, namely stroke volume, mean systolic ejection rate, mean left ventricular systolic pressure, left ventricular minute work index, and left ventricular efficiency index increased considerably. Initial exercise tests revealed progressive chest pain and up to 6 mm ST-T depression during performance of 300 KPM/min. The blood pressure of 130/80 did not rise at all during exercise. Nitroglycerin enabled him to exercise at 450 KPM/min for six minutes, and for one to two minutes at 600 KPM/min, at which level his abnormalities recurred.

This subject was monitored by ECG for the entire year's program of conditioning. Initially he exercised on the bicycle ergometer, with no change in his ECG or blood pressure responses. Following this he was retested on many occasions with a variety of drugs, and placed on isosorbide dinitrate, 20 mg six times a day, and propranolol, 40 mg twice a day for the remainder of the training year. The subject adherred faithfully to the training plan for three hours each week, and exercised for forty to fifty minutes at peak loads of 600 KPM/min for two to six minutes. He was able eventually to jog slowly four to five laps at a time. Chest pain appeared regularly on the fourth lap and reached 2+ by the end of the fifth lap. Recreational activity was carried out in a swimming pool. On a number of occasions medication was discontinued for three days, and the subject was retested (Fig. 8-17). In the absence of medication there was no improvement in WL_{120} during the year. On the other hand, the drugs improved his work performance promptly and reproducibly. Nitroglycerin, added to the other drugs, produced additional improvement. His blood pressure increased on rare occasions only, with effort.

At any given work load nitroglycerin always produced a *decrease* in the heart rate which paralleled the decrease in ST-T segment depression, rather than the usual tachycardia which was produced in the first subject.

PATIENT G.S.

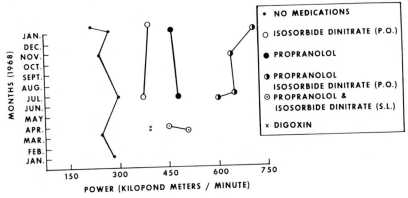

Figure 8-17. WL_{120} has been calculated from multiple standard exercise tests during one year of physical training. The medications indicated were administered for at least two days prior to testing. Propranol and isosorbide dinitrate were discontinued three days prior to testing without medications and five days prior to cardiac catherization. The series of four effort tests administered in January 1969 were conducted under "double-blind" conditions for each of the drugs. Digoxin was discontinued at least two weeks prior to further tests.

Figure 8-18 shows the effects of drugs on ECG ST-T depression. This effect followed the same pattern as did WL_{120}. The ECG and blood pressure responses at all times determined the maximal extent of effort.

Peripheral venous lactate levels during exercise did not rise significantly during maximally attainable exercise (300 KPM/min). However, with each of the drugs, the rise in venous lactate corresponded to the additional severity of work which the subject was afforded and paralleled improvements in heart rate and ECG response (Fig. 8-19).

This case is enigmatic in many ways. The significance of the apparent paradox between improvements in myocardial function and lack of change in work tolerance remains unknown. The drugs in some unknown way may have prevented the usual manifestations of physical training from appearing. It is not likely that the long-term

PATIENT G.S.

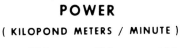

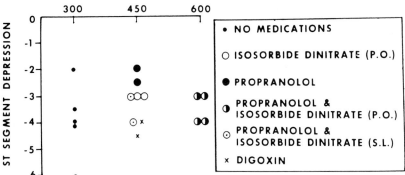

ECG CHANGES AT HIGHEST ATTAINABLE EFFORT LEVEL

Figure 8-18. ST segment measurements were all made from the same ECG lead (V₄ minus head), during the last five seconds of the exercise periods, during effort tests throughout a year of conditioning as represented in Figure 8-17.

use of isosorbide dinitrate and particularly propranolol were responsible for the improvements seen in myocardial function. The effects of propranolol on myocardial function during exercise are different from those found here (67). Other investigators have found variable effects of propranolol on exercise performance in subjects with angina pectoris (68, 69). In any event it is clear that propranolol and isosorbide dinitrate did not facilitate physical training, as determined by heart rate, blood pressure, and ECG responses to effort while no medications were being administered, even though they improved physical performance considerably, and even though peripheral lactate responses to effort indicated that conditions for training were present. Controlled studies must be carried out to determine the role of medications as an adjunct to the physical training of subjects with severe myocardial impairment.

In retrospect the first subject would have been a good candidate

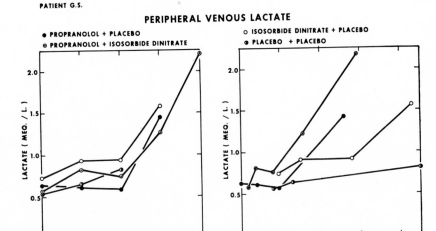

Figure 8-19. In this double blind study, peripheral venous lactate levels corresponded to the level of effort performed regardless of the medications used. As work performance improved and heart rate response to exercise decreased on each of the medications, peripheral venous lactate rose. Exercise conditions denoted by ⊙ were typical of those employed in physical training.

for physical training in an adequate clinical training center. The second subject would have to be considered, clinically, a poor training risk on the basis of his initially abnormal blood pressure response to effort and his subsequent lack of improvement after a short period of initial training before drugs were instituted. His inability to increase systolic blood pressure in response to effort may have been the most pertinent determinant in excluding him from a clinical training program. A third subject, who had severe angina and localized obstruction of the left anterior descending coronary artery, responded in a similar manner to the second subject: i.e. significant increase in work performance with medications, but only slight improvement when they were withdrawn. There was no evidence that drugs facilitated physical training, although parameters of myocardial function showed improvement following withdrawal of medications.

The comparison of the above subjects emphasizes that the ability to attain fitness may not be influenced primarily by the severity of anatomic arterial narrowing alone, as evaluated by cineangiography, but by these anatomic considerations in conjuction with myocardial function. Thus, a subject with slight myocardial damage might be expected to show more improvement with training than one with more myocardial damage even though the former had more extensive stenosis of the coronary arteries. Poor mechanical function is reflected indirectly in the response of the systolic blood pressure to exercise more than in other clinical parameters. ECG abnormalities would not be expected to reflect myocardial contractile function and do not necessarily correlate with severity of coronary arterial disease. Although important, ECG improvement is not helpful in assessing myocardial mechanical response to effort. Other clinical means of assessing this response must be employed (in addition to blood pressure, signs of inadequate cardiac output, and/or transient congestive heart failure).

Lipid and Glucose Metabolism

One of the major areas of dispute has been whether physical fitness per se affects cholesterol metabolism (70-93). Some of the difficulty in determining this conclusively relates to the problem of isolating exercise as a solitary variable. Most workers, who have found that physical training reduces serum cholesterol, have failed to exclude adequately diet and/or weight change as important influences. Well designed studies have, to the best of our knowledge, been carried out primarily in noncoronary subjects, and in young adult populations. In the CVAH study eleven subjects underwent C_{14} radioactive cholesterol turnover studies. Eight subjects underwent physical training, and three did not. Weight fluctuations did not exceed $\pm$ 2.5 pounds. Dietary diaries were kept for random three-day periods every three weeks for one year.* Weekly fasting serum samples were obtained for cholesterol ester fatty acids. Red blood cell samples were obtained for RBC fatty acids. Adipose tissue biopsy was obtained before and after training (a 9-month to twelve-month interval). The results available at this time relate to cholesterol turnover. There was no consistent difference in cholesterol turnover between trained and nontrained subjects nor between cholesterol turnover before and after the training period, at various levels of serum cholesterol.

Figure 8-20 shows a typical subject response. Cholesterol specific

---

* Under the direction of Dr. H. Houser, Case Western Reserve University, Department of Preventive Medicine.

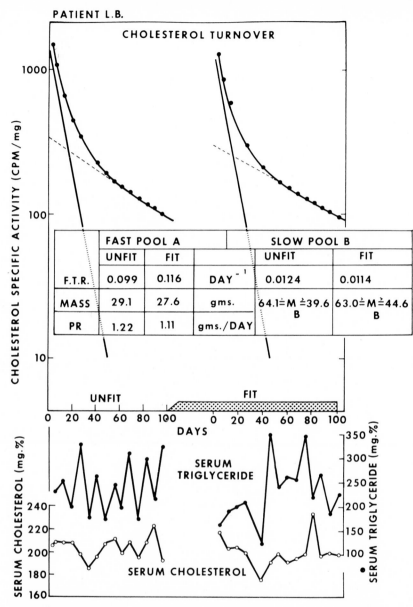

Figure 8-20. Example of cholesterol turnover and serum triglyceride and cholesterol levels determined weekly after an overnight fast before and after physical training. Standard deviation of duplicate samples equalled 1.32 mg% for cholesterol and 2.35 mg% for triglyceride determinations. The weekly variation of triglyceride levels was considerable, with no mean change. Cholesterol turnover and calculated pool characteristics remained unchanged. F. T. R. = fractional turnover rate. PR = production rate. The mass of pool B is calculated within arbitrary limits in accordance with a two-pool model.

activity curves conformed to a "two-pool model" whereby cholesterol turns over more rapidly in a pool thought to consist largely of serum, RBC, liver, lung, spleen, and kidney, and more slowly in a second pool consisting of other tissues. The percent of cholesterol leaving each pool (FTR $\times$ 100) did not change appreciably. The calculated quantity of cholesterol in each of the two pools (Mass) and the total body turnover rate (PR), assuming a steady state, did not vary appreciably. These data support the concept that fitness per se does not significantly influence overall cholesterol metabolism.

Regular exercise in the absence of weight change is associated with decrease in fat fold thickness (94). Although this was not studied in the CVAH subjects, many reported a decreasing belt size. Physical training might be expected to increase muscle mass and could be associated with shifts within the "slow" cholesterol pool without necessarily affecting its size or overall dynamics.

In contrast, in the CWRU-JCC study where a multifactoral approach was used, serum cholesterol levels obtained before and after physical training showed a reduction from 263 mg% to 242 mg%. This reduction reflects generally the reductions which are to be found in the literature. They are modest and do not exceed reductions obtained by diet alone. It is important to note that serum cholesterol reductions *can* be affected on a large scale with the use of dietary counselling at a community center.

Serum triglyceride levels have been found to decline acutely following a single exercise task of several hours duration (95). Holloszy has found reduction in serum triglycerides following physical training in sedentary normal middle-aged males (85). However, Mann *et al.*, in a well-designed study, showed no change (91). Weekly twelve-hour fasting triglyceride levels in our study fluctuated widely and did not change appreciably with physical training. Figure 8-20 shows one example. In addition, seventeen ASHD subjects underwent triglyceride turnover studies before and after physical training as a relative measure of the rate at which newly formed triglyceride is removed from the serum. Fourteen subjects physically trained, and three remained as untrained controls.

Turnover studies were carried out with the use of glycerol-H_3 and calculated from the specific activity of triglyceride glycerol in the very low density serum lipoprotein (96). There was no consistent change in triglyceride turnover following training.

Definite differences exist between this study and that of Holloszy's (86) in pretraining and posttraining fitness levels, and in other factors. Although the evidence for severe prolonged exertion causing reductions in serum triglyceride levels appears sound, the question remains as to the significance of this phenomenon in subjects whose relative fitness levels are comparatively modest. Under these latter circumstances, our studies did not show a significant reduction of serum triglycerides nor consistent change in triglyceride turnover in the very low density serum lipoproteins, which can be attributed to physical training.

Physical reconditioning probably does not influence glucose toler-

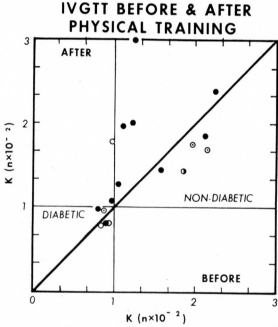

Figure 8-21. Intravenous glucose tolerance did not change with physical training.

ance in the subject with noninsulin dependent mild "chemical" diabetes. Six subjects at the CVAH demonstrated intolerance to intravenously administered glucose. There was no change in five of these following training. The sixth subject became more tolerant to glucose administration. Similarly, eight non-diabetic subjects showed no consistent change in their glucose tolerance following physical training. None developed abnormal K values (Fig. 8-21). Our data are in accord with those of two other studies of the intravenous (91) and oral glucose tolerance (97) and are divergent from the report of Davidson *et al.* which showed that the oral glucose tolerance was altered in the direction of diabetes (98).

Our findings do not suggest that physical training has no effect whatsoever on carbohydrate metabolism. In this regard, clinicians agree that the insulin requirement of insulin-dependent diabetic patients diminishes during increased physical activity. The reason for this is not known. It appears, though, that whatever relationships exist between physical fitness and carbohydrate metabolism, they have not become apparent with the use of clinical glucose tolerance tests.

DISCUSSION

Benefits

Prior to entering a training program subjects must be informed about the benefits and risks of such participation. In order to give informed consent, the subject should be provided with a review of the effects of training and fitness on cardiovascular function, potential benefits and risks, and of the nature of his commitment to such a program, in a fashion which is comprehensible to him. As the result of the practices of intake of subjects into our studies, we have developed a brochure which explains in detail, in a simple question-and-answer form, the studies which were undertaken. A brochure of similar format can be composed by altering the informational content to fit the needs of any particular study or training program. It should make very clear the limitations of a physical training facility and the importance of other aids, such as dietetic and psychological counselling and where they may be obtained. In addition, such a document should make clear the role and risks of exercise, in keeping with the aims of the Helsinki Declaration.

It is occasionally tempting to endow a physical reconditioning program with unrealistic health-promoting claims. One must be cautious not to exceed the limits of firm data in describing such programs. For example, numerous retrospective studies have shown that physically active subjects have a lower morbidity and mortality from myocardial infarction than those in sedentary occupations. This conclusion is reasonably firm, even if it is found in the future that such benefits are caused by an associated factor other than exercise per se. As yet large *controlled* prospective studies of the effects of enhanced physical fitness on mortality and morbidity of habitually inactive subjects have not been made. Nonetheless, in the absence of such definitive studies we can advocate physical fitness enhancement on the basis of the *likelihood* of reducing a risk factor. If one accepts physical activity as a necessary ingredient in daily living, it is justified to recommend strongly properly supervised physical training to ASHD subjects as well as to apparently normal middle-aged men, with the hope of improving general function in daily activity and promoting a feeling of well-being. These are good reasons to train. However caution must be taken to guard against increased risk by improper exercise. With proper screening and adequately supervised physical activity there has been and should be no increase in the mortality associated with ASHD. The present studies and epidemiological data strongly suggest that supervised physical training is not detrimental. One cannot claim at the present time that fitness will *extend* life or *prevent* a heart attack, although we certainly hope that it will. Nor can one claim that fitness, by itself, will reduce serum lipids in a meaningful way, or improve glucose tolerance, or cause significant weight reduction. Reduction of the other risk factors undertaken in conjunction with physical fitness should constitute optimal therapy.

In special uncontrolled circumstances sudden exhaustive effort may precipitate acute myocardial infarction or sudden death. This possibility *must* be included in describing a program.

Potential Hazards

The most important cause of increased risk in our opinion is inappropriate overactivity because of unsupervised sudden exertion.

Recently a number of deaths have been reported in subjects undergoing currently popular "do-it-yourself" jogging programs (99). The NCP subject, in whom the potentiality for severe coronary disease is not recognized, is particularly vulnerable in unsupervised programs. The high incidence of death in the natural course of ASHD regardless of the level of physical activity (61) makes it impossible to exclude *all* deaths from any regimen. It would therefore be unreasonable to discontinue programs where the occurrence of death and myocardial infarction is not increased. Instead, specific steps must be taken to educate subjects and professional staffs in the proper use of this modality (100).

In supervised exercise programs it would appear that the greatest hazard might likewise lie in the subject's overactivity, above and beyond that which is appropriate for him at any given time. Associated with this hazard are potential errors in the exercise prescription which call for levels of activity which are inappropriately excessive. This factor is controllable with appropriate supervision of the training sessions. On the other hand in the initial training period, many subjects experience a marked feeling of well-being far in excess of the actual improvement in their fitness. At this time, these participants are especially vulnerable to the indiscretion of exceeding their training prescriptions.

Untoward circumstances have been related to premonitory feelings of weakness, inappropriately severe fatigue, and transitory confusion before, during, and after exercise sessions. Such symptoms are assumed to be insignificant and are usually not reported by the average participant (101). The milieu of a reconditioning program should be such that encourages the participants reporting "odd" feelings *prior to exercise* or as soon as possible during sessions. At that time, identification of a hitherto undetected arrhythmia or of a newly developing one may be life-saving. In addition, exercise should probably be postponed following a night of poor or little sleep, or after an unusually stressful day. A period of rest and relaxation following the exercise session is advisable. It must be continually kept in mind that even in a training program cardiovascular difficulties associated with exercise do not occur only in known ASHD subjects. NCP and "normal" subjects are at risk as well (102), as they are in the course of their usual daily life. Participants in a training program must be exhorted to follow their exercise prescriptions faithfully and to report any new symptoms.

During or after physical activity ventricular arrhythmias may occur suddenly, either as single extrasystoles, frequently spaced regularly between every one to five or six sinus beats, or in paroxysms of two or more consecutive ectopic beats. These may be accompanied by odd chest sensations such as a "thump" (which may represent the increased cardiac activity in the postextrasystolic beat), by a feeling that the heart "skipped a beat," or in the extreme case, by light-headedness and syncope.

Newly appearing single extrasystoles during exercise are warnings to stop and rest. Some "normal" as well as ASHD subjects have isolated ventricular extrasystoles at rest. These beats usually do not arise at dangerous points in ventricular recovery cycle (at the peak of the ECG T wave), when they would be likely to trigger ventricular fibrillation. When innocuous, in most cases they disappear once exercise has been started. There seems to be no cause for undue concern under these circumstances. However, where ventricular extrasystoles regularly increase with exercise, or appear at the peak of the T wave of the preceding beat, they must be treated either with modification of the exercise prescription, and/or with antiarrhythmic drugs. Paroxysms or runs of ventricular extrasystoles during severe exercise may commence without advance notice and are to be considered extremely dangerous!

In the CVAH study new ventricular arrhythmias have served as an indication to terminate the current exercise session. If the arrhythmia disappeared promptly an exercise test was repeated the following day. If the arrhythmia recurred at work loads which the subject had previously tolerated, exercise was witheld for three to seven days in order to detect any change in the clinical state. If no complications appeared, testing and exercise was resumed at a lower level. If a ventricular arrhythmia appeared at a level of exercise below that which the subject had tolerated in the past, and if it recurred similarly during the second test on the following day, exercise was reduced below this level. In one subject, antiarrhythmic drugs were used. At the CVAH, ventricular arrhythmias have occurred

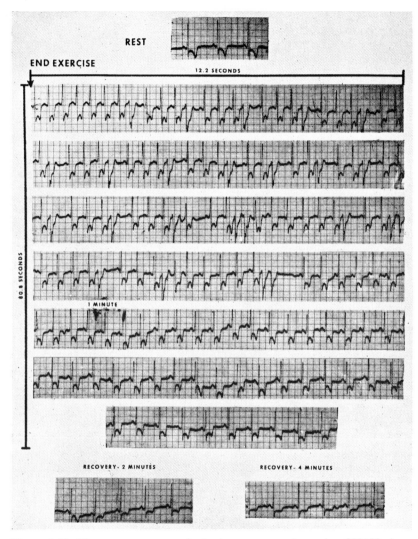

Figure 8-22. The most severe arrhythmia encountered at the CVAH, in a subject with severe angina after ten months of physical training. This sequence was recorded following seven laps of jogging (this subject usually jogs five laps at a time). ST-T displacement is "usual" for this subject. The ventricular arrhythmia never occurred at less prolonged exercise.

infrequently. The worst has been paroxysms of two ventricular beats, most often during the first minute of recovery following which they have invariably completely disappeared (Fig. 8-22). To date they have not been reproducible and have not recurred on subsequent testing. We have tentatively concluded that although isolated instances of arrhythmia need not necessarily herald a change in the clinical condition of the subject, they require close observation.

Ventricular arrhythmias must be regarded as being serious because they may be harbingers of fatal complications, ventricular fibrillation, or cardiac arrest. We have provided each exercise area with readily available resuscitation equipment (drugs, airway, bag respirator, and defibrillator) and personnel trained in the technique of resuscitation.

Practical Application of Initial Evaluation

The quality and relevence of the initial evaluation is very important. It is likewise essential that the evaluation be carried out in as prompt and practical way as possible. In our opinion histories and cardiac-oriented physical examinations should be performed at the training facility. Histories can be obtained with the use of question forms specifically designed for the purpose, administered by non-medical personnel, completed largely by the subjects without supervision, and evaluated by the attending physician. The physician can review the history with the subject at the time of the physical examination. Standard question forms are used in order to save time and effort on the part of the program staff. However, such a device does not substitute for the interpersonal relationship which must develop early between the staff and subjects in order to carry out the program successfully. The physical examination as well as the history provide means of identifying clinical conditions which might preclude exercise testing, such as congestive heart failure. Resting 12 lead ECGs and serum lipids should be obtained in all subjects.

Exercise testing must be standard, informative, and as brief as possible. For this reason we have instituted an abbreviated bicycle ergometer test, and methods for carrying out multiple tests simultaneously, with a minimum of personnel and a maximum of centralized supervision. These have been described above. There is a limit beyond which further abbreviation of testing procedures sacrifices much informative value, and becomes potentially more risky. The mode of testing (bicycle, treadmill, etc.) is not a primary concern. However, in our opinion, features of the testing procedure should include multiple progressive work loads for three or more minutes duration, intervening rest periods, intermittent monitoring of the ECG and blood pressure, and continuous monitoring of the heart rate of the subjects being tested. Testing personnel should be able to recognize ECG ST-T displacement, the pattern of ventricular arrhythmias, and alterations in QRS configuration and in the relationship between atrial and ventricular depolarization. In addition, they should be familiar with normal responses to testing and the recognition of the more frequently encountered potential problems, such as inappropriate blood pressure responses and postexercise bradycardia. In our experience these techniques can be taught to, and proficiently practiced by, nonphysicians in the presence of adequate medical supervision. Programmed periodic teaching sessions can be carried out in the same fashion as is currently being done in coronary care units throughout the country.

Target Levels for Training in the Absence of "Strain"

Exercise prescriptions are determined largely by the heart rate and ECG response to the initial effort test. The purpose of the initial exercise test is to determine the target level for training and to provide a basis for future comparative fitness measurements. Figure 8-23 depicts principles of determining this target level. In the absence of "strain" (abnormal response to exercise) our subjects exercised at an average of 60 to 70 percent of their maximal aerobic power. This level is equivalent to 70 to 85 percent of the age adjusted maximal heart rate respectively: that is, average exercise to 70 percent and peak exercise of short duration to 85 percent of age adjusted maximal heart rate.

The age adjustment consists of a decrease of approximately six beats per minute per five years of life from a maximal heart rate of 200 beats per minute at age 25.* For example:

---

* This value was calculated from a graph constructed by Samuel M. Fox, III, M.D.

Age (Years)	Age Adjusted Max H.R.	Target H.R.	
		85% MHR	70% MHR
35	188	160	132
45	176	149	123
55	164	140	115
% Max O_2 Uptake	100%	78%	52%

TARGET LEVELS FOR TRAINING

In Absence of "Strain"

60% to 70% of maximal aerobic power (MAP).

Heart rate (HR) equivalent to 60% to 70% MAP.

Age adjusted maximal heart rate (MHR)-

Average expenditure 70% of MHR.

Peak expenditure to 85% of MHR.

In Symptomatic Subjects

Heart rate

Less than that which produces ECG changes (marked ST-T displacement, ectopic activity)

Inappropriate blood pressure responses

Symptoms and signs (severe pain, dyspnea, confusion)

Symptoms

Pain (intensity, distribution and sequence)

Dyspnea

Central nervous system symptoms

Figure 8-23. Guideline for training targets.

Energy expenditure estimations can be expressed also in approximate terms of percent maximal oxygen uptake, kilocalories (kcal), or metabolic units (METS), where

1 MET = O_2 uptake at rest (not basal)

1 MET = approximately 4 ml O_2/kg body weight/min (B.W./min).

1 kcal = 200 ml O_2 uptake

For example, calculating for a 75 kg man:

4 ml O_2 × 75 Kg = 300 ml O_2/min = 1.5 kcal = 1 MET

If maximal O_2 uptake = 2.25 l, O_2/min,

$$\frac{2.25 \text{ l}}{75 \text{ kg}} = 30 \text{ ml } O_2/\text{kg B.W./min} = 7.5 \text{ METS}$$

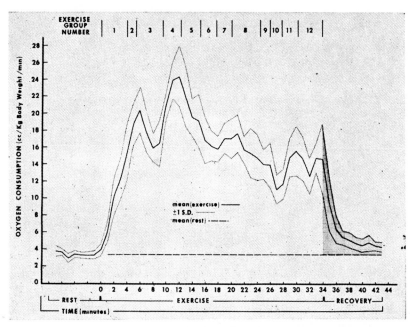

Figure 8-24. Oxygen cost of consecutively performed calisthenics done routinely in the CWRU-FCC study. Exercise numbers signify performance of the following exercises: (1) shoulder exercises, standing, warm-up; (2) hops, walk steps; (3) arm sweeps, standing; (4) hops, sailor's hornpipe; (5) body bends; (6) leg exercises, supine; (7) leg-arm-hip exercise, sitting on floor; (8) leg exercises, lying on side; (9) leg exercises, bicycle movements, supine; (10)sit-ups; (11) push-ups; and (12) shoulder exercises, standing, cool off.

In the CWRU-JCC study a predetermined sequence of calisthenics of measured oxygen cost was utilized (Fig. 8-24): at peak exercise 22-26 ml O_2/kg B.W./min (5.4-6.5 METS). At average exercise O_2 uptake was 14-18 ml O_2/kg B.W./min (3.5-4.5 METS). For a 75 kg man with maximal oxygen uptake of 2.25 1/min (30 mlO_2/kg B.W./min) the calisthenics required were from 73 to 87 percent and 47-60 percent of maximal oxygen uptake, respectively, and compared closely with the above recommended mean of 78 percent and 52 percent.

Likewise the average heart rate response to calesthenics (120 beats/min) approximated the recommended 70 percent of age adjusted maximal heart rates. After physical training, heart rates decreased uniformly as expected (Fig. 8-25).

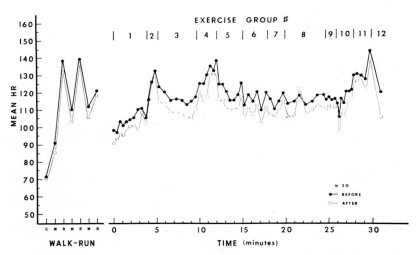

Figure 8-25. Average heart rates of walk-run sequences (W = walk, R = run, C = control) and of consecutively performed calisthenics done routinely in the CWRU-JCC study.

The electrocardiograms of twenty subjects (average age 48 yrs) were tele-metered before (solid lines) and several months after (dotted lines) participation in the program. Note that the average heart rate was almost 120 beats per minute, representing 70 percent of their predicted maximal heart rate. Exercise numbers signify performance of the following exercises: (1) shoulder exercises, standing, warm-up; (2) hops, walk steps; (3) arm sweeps, standing; (4) hops, sailor's hornpipe; (5) body bends; (6) leg exercises, supine; (7) leg-arm-hip exercise, sitting on floor; (8) leg exercises, lying on side; (9) leg exercises, bicycle movements, supine; (10) sit-ups; (11) push-ups; and (12) shoulder exercises, standing, cool off.

The goal of physical training is to attain physical fitness conducive to good cardiovascular function and good health. The attainment of the desired level of fitness should occur in orderly fashion usually at a *restrained* rate of progress. Competition with others should be singularly avoided. Initially the goal for improvement should be directed toward the development of self-confidence and appreciation of improvements and proficiency of performance (body motions, coordination, etc.). Only later should the subject compete with himself by increasing the pace or duration of his activity. Target levels for training, as calculated and defined above, should be used only as guidelines. These levels must be adjusted for each subject individually, with the aid of clinical observations and response to the initial effort test, to arrive at an "actual" target level. This "actual" target level may vary somewhat from day to day depending on daily fluctuations in the subject's other activities. There is good rationale for making such a calculation, inasmuch as bicycle ergometers are now becoming available for home use, which are calibrated in units of absolute power (KPM/min) and which display heart rate response.* These units are also fitted with sound systems which indicate to the subjects the relation of their heart rates to a preset target rate. In the future it should be quite feasible to prescribe precise practical exercise programs for large groups of people.

Target for Training in the Presence of "Strain"

The above general remarks firmly apply to subjects with abnormal exercise responses, as well as to those with normal responses. The prescription of exercise for abnormal responders differs according to the criteria outlined in Figure 8-23. The target level for training is defined as that level at which or below which progressive abnormalities occur. The latter includes the appearance of frequent ventricular premature beats of tachycardia, atrioventricular conduction defects, marked ST-T displacement (3 mm or more, less if associated with severe angina pectoris or its equivalent), disproportionate blood pressure responses (too high or too low, failure to increase blood pressure with higher work loads), central nervous system symptoms of confusion, incoordination, chest pain with increasing radiation and severity, and excessive dyspnea.

Targets for training subjects with "strain" are adjustable and may be influenced by certain medications which, in some circumstances, have been shown to increase work load performance (nitroglycerin, isosorbide dinitrate, and propanolol). These drugs can be particularly helpful in some symptomatic subjects in their activities of early living. However, their usefulness as adjuncts to physical training in asymptomatic as well as symptomatic ASHD subjects has yet to be determined. The present pilot studies indicate that the answer

---

* Manufactured by Lifecycle, Inc., 1006 Shary Circle, Concord, California, 94520, and Schwinn Bicycle Co., 1856 North Kostner Ave., Chicago, Illinois, 60639.

to this question may be complex. At present nitroglycerin is the only drug which can be recommended without reservation in appropriate subjects.

Physical Training

Following the initial evaluation, normal subjects who have no evidence of coronary proneness or ASHD may start immediately in a training program at appropriate fitness levels. Subjects with varying degrees of coronary proneness, likewise, may enter training at somewhat more restricted levels.

The CWRU-JCC and CVAH experiences indicate that optimal circumstances of physical training of the symptomatic ASHD subject can be approached only if ECG monitoring is employed in the early training period. Close supervision is essential until the subject and the physician have been educated as to the pattern, progression, and regression of abnormalities. When monitoring is not feasible, training activities should be lighter than the level performed on frequent monitored ergometer tests, and the subjects should rest with the appearance of symptoms. Three to ten subjects can be monitored at one time during the initial training period of two to four weeks. Longer monitoring may be needed for severely symptomatic subjects. The most critical ingredient in training subjects with severe ASHD is highly skilled supervision.

Patterns of exercise in the symptomatic subject do not differ greatly from those used in nonsymptomatic subjects except for the factors which determine peak severity: for nonsymptomatic subjects with normal response to exercise tests, a predetermined heart rate, and for abnormal responders, the level at which progressive abnormality occurs.

Representative examples of the patterns of exercise for symptomatic subjects are shown in Figures 8-26 and 8-27. Interval training with short bouts of higher work loads, interspersed with longer duration lighter work loads and intermittent rest periods, has been most satisfactory (Fig. 8-26). Unsatisfactory patterns of exercise are shown in Figure 8-27. In the upper two rows the work load is too large and prolonged and can lead to severe symptoms of fatigue, anxiety and perhaps undue risk. In the lower two rows the magni-

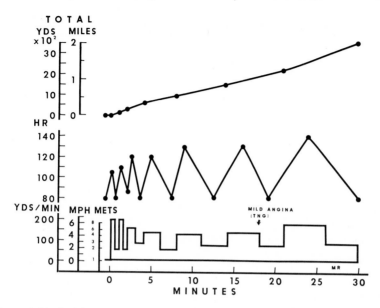

Figure 8-26. Satisfactory pattern of exercise to improve both endurance and intensity of performance in the symptomatic ASHD subject. (See text.)

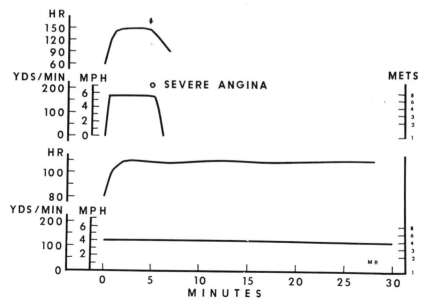

Figure 8-27. Two patterns of exercise which are not satisfactory. (See text.)

tude of work load is small. When repeated session after session, this exercise pattern might be expected to increase endurance somewhat but not to increase work tolerance. Sustained effort of low magnitude is important either in conjunction with supervised training, or alone, for subjects who are unsuitable for training. Such subjects may take long leisurely walks when the outdoor temperature is moderate.

Bed rest for prolonged periods leads to significant changes in cardiovascular function (103). As a safety precaution in both NCP and ASHD subjects, it is recommended that the resumption of physical training following bed rest, even for a few days, be modified. In such an instance, a subject should perform minimal exercise in the first session and progress up the scale of his original exercise prescriptions, abbreviating the periods of time at each level. In so doing, he should probably reach his former level in a time period relative to his period of inactivity. In the absence of definitive data on this question, the following "rule of thumb" has been used at the CVAH: A subject would achieve his previous fitness level in not less than one session per bedridden day up to three bedridden days, and not less than one session per bedridden day plus four to five extra sessions, for four to fifteen days of confinement (assuming three sessions per week) provided that the period of ambulatory convalescence following relative bedrest is not excessive. For example, if a subject were confined to bed for six days, with three subsequent days of ambulatory convalescence, he would resume training at a low level, and progress to former fitness gradually, in a minimum of ten sessions or approximately three weeks 1 session $\times$ 6 bedridden days $+$ 4 extra sessions). Longer periods of bedrest or protracted ambulatory convalescence probably necessitate retraining from the initial fitness level, with a prescription similar to that which the subject originally followed. We feel that the guidelines described here are particularly necessary for those subjects who are receiving medications which alter the heart rate response. In such subjects it might be difficult to use the heart rate to determine accurately appropriate retraining work loads.

Proscriptions of Potential Hazards

Some factors or practices frequently associated with physical training sessions should be specifically prohibited and cautioned against, both for NCP and ASHD subjects:

1. Dry or wet "hot" rooms or towels.
2. Cold or very hot showers, before or immediately after training sessions.
3. Iced or very hot drinks, or alcoholic beverages.
4. Passing quickly from a warm locker room into winter weather while still perspiring.
5. Ingestion of large meals either less than two hours before or within one hour following active exercise.
6. Smoking, at all times, but particularly while dressing after exercise.
7. The ingestion of coffee before or after exercise.

The above features are important because they constitute additional stresses to the cardiovascular systems. It is well known that thermal stress (extremes of heat or cold) can evoke considerable strain in man. Sudden death during snow shovelling is due to a combination of the effects of cold exposure and sudden severe effort in an unconditioned subject. The ingestion of fluids at extreme temperatures is known to produce cardiac arrhythmias. Large meals tend to divert a greater portion of the cardiac output to mesenteric vascular beds. Such meals can also cause ECG changes in ASHD subjects. Other items specific to individual training facilities should be sought and added to the above list.

Adherence

In the CWRU-JCC study fitness was enhanced in direct relation to adherence. Figure 8-10 shows that improvement occurred only in those who attended approximately two exercise sessions or more a week. Attendance of more than five to six exercise sessions per month did not confer greater ECG benefit and conferred only slightly increased benefit in level of fitness. From these data it might be inferred that truly high degrees of fitness (of champion magnitude) are *not* needed in order to gain significant cardiac benefits from an exercise program. (This opinion is shared by other workers.) Furthermore, since these data reflect varied levels of fitness achievement, it is entirely possible that adherence rather than level of training is a more important clinical index of relative benefit, as far as the participating subjects are concerned. In a community conditioning program it would be justified, if not desirable, to adopt a policy of

encouragement and reward on the basis of adherence and attendance
to the program and to the individual exercise prescriptions, even if
the magnitude of effort was less than "optimally" strenuous. Initial
emphasis upon attendance and participation instead of performance
achievement has several advantages. Such an orientation might:

1. Support a noncompetitive attitude on the part of the supervising personnel and subjects.
2. Encourage more restraint to sudden severe effort by those subjects who ordinarily might exceed the exercise prescription early
   in training when they have achieved a feeling of well-being.
3. Encourage less competitive people in the community to join
   fitness programs.
4. Make it possible to employ individual types of training regimens
   which can be geared to train subjects for specific exertional
   tasks required by their individual vocational and social pattern
   of life activities, rather than encouraging uniform "assembly
   line" type of physical training progress which might tend to
   stratify subjects on the basis of performance or prowess.

Behavioral Aspects of Training

There is little doubt that in many subjects physical training along
with the environment of a training facility and other adjunctive
measures may contribute significantly to the subject's "quality of
life." Subjects in a training program frequently report that they
are better able to organize and execute their occupational responsibilities, that they have suddenly found ways of providing more free
time for relaxation, and that their interpersonal relationships have
improved. Reduction of anxiety towards their disease undoubtedly
plays an important part. However, in addition, several of our subjects have claimed that they have reviewed their entire lifes' pattern.
Some of the far reaching decisions which they have made suggest
that this may indeed be true. In a few cases, the advent of physical
conditioning has been followed by major changes in occupation toward more satisfying and less emotionally demanding work.

The clinical observation has been made that myocardial infarct
frequently is preceded by severe emotional stress. Gruen has found a
greater occurrence of occupational and marital interpersonal diffi-

culties in ASHD subjects than in non-ASHD subjects (104). Whether or not a causal relationship exists between responses to environmental stress and ASHD, these experiences furnish clues that ASHD subjects and perhaps NCP subjects share an altered environmental response, or an altered personal environment, which may be modified in some unknown way by a conditioning program.

Unfortunately it is more difficult to quantitate the responses to environmental stresses than other physiological states. Psychological testing recognizes the need for such a measurement, but is still an inadequate tool to describe accurately emotional responses to environmental stress and their mediation. Biological and emotional needs and satisfactions are not necessarily interdependent, yet both apply to physical fitness in the ASHD subject. Investigation in this area is still rudimentary. P. V. Simonov states that "the investigation of physiological mechanisms of emotion has meaning not only in relation to man's social problems, but also for practical matters such as engineering, pedagogy, art, sport, medicine, and psychoneurology. This is one of the most important fields of modern research in the physiology of higher nervous activity" (105).

Role of the Spouse

In programs where wives are interviewed periodically along with their husbands, the common experiences can frequently promote greater mutual understanding of the participants clinical state. This is desirable, since the participant's health problems affect his entire family, and since sharing of such experiences frequently reduces covert anxieties in each spouse. The wife can become instrumental in the subject's management by providing a stabilizing influence to help maintain fitness or prevent her husband's enthusiasm from converting an exercise program into a fad, which occasionally occurs. In addition, since dietary changes invariably enter into the wife's domain, her participation and education are essential. Furthermore, in our experience, unless some direct contact is maintained with the wife, whereby she is informed of his progress, an uncomfortable situation frequently arises in which the subject is torn between the program staff's recommendations to increase the level of training and the wife's understandable efforts to restrain her husband's activity.

It is important that she develop confidence in her husband's ability to recognize his safe limits and act accordingly, since realistically he is the only one who is in a position to exert effective judgment. Likewise, the husband may need help to understand his wife's reasonable concern about his health and physical training. He must be encouraged to keep her informed of his progress. A positive attitude of the wife enhances her husband's motivation and adherence to the physical training program.

The fact that no mention has been made of physical training of NCP or ASHD women does not imply that this subject is less important. Similar principles and methods undoubtedly will apply.

Role of the Physical Educators

Physical training is but one part of the total management of the ASHD subject. The subject's medical management must at all times remain completely under the control of his private physician. Physical educators and cardiologists conducting training programs should reinforce measures of the private physician to establish good health practices. They must maintain close communication with the private physician to report his patient's response to the training program. Because of the frequent contacts between the subjects and the supervisory personnel, special attention must be directed towards avoiding an alienation of the private physician. His role must not be usurped in any way.

The above discussion does not minimize the responsibility assumed, knowingly or unknowingly, by anyone who undertakes to train ASHD and/or normal subjects. It is desirable to promote a positive outlook in the subjects and an attitude that their physical training is meant to improve their lives in general rather than to treat specifically an affliction. However, equally true is the fact that supervised physical training *is* a *medical* intervention in ASHD subjects which carries with it the legal and professional responsibilities of medical and health practices.

The nature of the therapy and the subject population require that the role of the physical educator be expanded to one which includes full active "membership" in the health professions. This should be implemented by instituting appropriate courses of study in his educational background, and by inviting his participation in the design as well as the implementation of reconditioning programs for ASHD subjects.

Program Design

It may be impractical to operate a service function in the same manner as one which is research oriented. However, since a large segment of our population falls into the NCP and ASHD groups, it is necessary to provide acceptable physical activity programs in which such subjects can participate with a maximum degree of safety. There are a number of possible approaches to designing a physical training program. Basically they all rely on the interaction of variables in personnel and facilities and the depth and proficiency of the initial evaluation.

For example, in a facility where ECG monitoring, physician supervision, and direct supervision during training sessions are not available, but where a prescribed regimen for training can be given on the basis of heart rate response to standard effort, unfit subjects over thirty years who are normal or only minimally coronary prone, by history, should be accepted. Minimal coronary proneness in this context refers to a male subject with only one of the coronary prone traits by history, such as smoking, overweight (not obese), or borderline hypertension. Marked obesity (more than 20% above the desirable weight is considered a relative contraindication. Subjects with a family history of coronary disease under the age of sixty arbitrarily are considered to be more than minimally coronary prone. The inclusion of a physician and ECG effort tests expands the scope of the training program to include NCP and ASHD subjects who show normal ECG response to standard progressive exercise, *provided that the training regimen does not require heart rates exceeding the highest heart rate reached on the exercise test.* Direct supervision of the training regimen in the form of an experienced physical educator watching and counselling the subjects during their activities plus a technician knowledgeable in ECG interpretation and/or a physician to monitor appropriate subjects during the early phases of physical training meet the requirements needed for a program for subjects with abnormal ECG responses to effort. The extent to which abnormal responders can be included thus depends upon the size and interests of the staff.

If physical training is to be offered to ASHD subjects, it might be advisable for each community to establish a facility specifically designed for the effort evaluation and initial training of these subjects. Such a facility could be patterned after or combined with work-classification clinics and "coronary clubs" which are operative in major cities. This is already being done in several cities in the USA and in Europe. Centers can be established to instruct physicians and allied health personnel. Following initial testing, adjustment of medications, and a four-week to eight-week period of training, these subjects could be gradually transferred to local community fitness facilities to continue activity at a slightly lower level than that achieved, under the guidance of participating physical educators. These subjects could be reevaluated at the evaluation center periodically, or as clinical conditions change. Initial training could consist of bicycling, calisthentics, jogging in place, and other activities available at the initial training center, which stress large muscle groups and permit simultaneous ECG monitoring. As training progresses *home exercise programs can in some instances be instituted at work levels slightly lower than those employed during training sessions.*

The current "state of the art" requires that data collection, collation, and analysis be built into the design of a reconditioning program. Simply obtained information may be very useful when compared with similarly obtained information from other centers. Data systems set up *in advance* are infinitely more valuable than those which are constructed in retrospect. The types of data gathered may be many and depend upon the scope of each training program. Information kept in a simple digital manner on master code sheets allows an immediate perusal of the subject population.

Research into the general and cardiovascular effects of physical training is in its infancy. As more attention becomes focused on environmental adaptation of subjects with various disease states, community service organizations become increasingly vital as laboratories. Conversely, safety procedures and new knowledge must be imparted to community facilities to keep them up to date and to insure the safest and most efficient use of their program. The scientist and the physical educator must therefore merge into a closely working team. Widespread uniform practical means must be adopted for the accumulation of important controlled data and dissemination of their analysis. This can best be done with the cooperation of organizations such as the YMCA and the American Heart Association, where cooperative protocols can be constructed and carried out on a national basis. The prototype for such studies has been well developed and is being employed by certain national and international organizations in the study of various medical problems and in aiding the operation of ongoing programs.

In paying specific attention to potential hazards and safety features of physical training programs, it is not the intention of this chapter to point out obstacles which make the operation of a program impractical. Quite the reverse! To recognize that a proper training program is difficult to achieve, is not to say that it is impossible, or in the long run, impractical. Although the initial investment may be large, the dividends are proportionate, and the maintenance costs far less.

Physical Training Versus Other Therapies

Physical training cannot be compared with other therapies for ASHD (other medical and surgical procedures) at this time. Medically, physical fitness is perhaps best thought of as being adjunctive to other therapies, to be used appropriately in conjuction with them, not in place of them. No treatment has yet been found which can prevent or reverse the underlying fat and fibrous tissue-containing arterial lesions of atherosclerosis. There is no good reason to believe at this time that exercise, or other current therapies will be found capable of achieving this result. However, it is hoped that exercise, and other current therapies can forestall and attenuate the appearance of progressively limiting clinical manifestations (such as "heart attack") and thereby prolong fruitful life. At this time our medical capability is limited to this goal, and we must make the most of it.

SUMMARY AND CONCLUSIONS

Experience in a large "fitness" feasibility study and a detailed small "pilot" study have provided some insights into practical requirements in the physical training of ASHD and NCP subjects. In addition some tentative conclusions have been drawn regarding relative risks and benefits of physical training relating to myocardial function, lipid and carbohydrate metabolism, and clinical and emotional aspects of the subjects. The following list of simplified guidelines might serve as a basis for the operation of community "fitness" programs for people who are at risk of developing coronary heart disease, and those who already suffer from it.

1. Fitness is relative and must be individualized.
2. It is desirable to promote enthusiasm but to discourage inter-participant competition and faddism.
3. The subject's spouse must be specifically included in the subject's training and counselling experience.
4. Subject's symptoms can be useful in assessing limitations in physical training. During the course of training subjects should undergo an educational process whereby they learn to become accurate clinical judges of their own energy expenditure and physical and cardiac abilities. This must be accomplished largely by experience with reassurance without preoccupation with somatic functions.
5. The type of large-muscle group dynamic exercise is not critical, but should relate to aptitude, interest, and specific limitations. Strenuous arm and isometric exercises should be avoided. A standard exercise procedure should be included as the initial task of each training sessions, during which the heart rate response and in appropriate subjects, the ECG response, are recorded.
6. Time taken to attain "fitness" is not critical. It will vary with adherence, medical problems, as well as the personality of each participant. Emphasis should be placed more on interest and attendance rather than on fitness achievement. The latter will occur *pari passu* if the subject adheres properly to a well planned exercise prescription.
7. In addition to identifying subjects with high coronary risk and with ASHD, screening procedures should aim to separate subjects into two overall groups:

A. In which the limiting factor to performance is untrained peripheral muscles or "unfit" oxygen transport system.

B. In which the limiting factor to performance is myocardial ischemia resulting from coronary heart disease.

(This implies the use of multilevel effort tests with ECG and blood pressure monitoring.)

Group A may train without monitoring but with a definite strict progressive regimen. Group B should be tested initially with and without medications (nitroglycerine, isosorbide dinitrate, or other medications as needed). As a minimum, the effects of nitroglycerin on the response to standard effort should be assessed. Propranolol is not yet approved for general use. If, and when it is approved, it should be administered cautiously only by physicians experienced in its use. Subjects should then be placed on the appropriate medication(s) in conjunction with physical exercise. Monitoring the initial period of physical training is essential. Subjects must show reproducibility of responses to effort, and upper safe limits must be established before monitoring can be discontinued.

8. Nitroglycerin in small doses (0.3 mg) may be used prophylactically and frequently by symptomatic subjects *and asymptomatic subjects* with ASHD both in the presence and absence of abnormal ECG responses to effort.

9. Physical training should be started slowly, allowing no less than two weeks for acclimatization to the regimen.

10. Training sessions should consist of

A. A period of "warm-up."

B. Endurance activity of moderate severity. (70% of maximal age-adjusted heart rate).

C. "Peak" activities of short duration approaching 85% of maximal heart rate or at the threshold of progressive symptoms or signs of myocardial ischemia.

D. Tapering-off exercises to avoid hypotension and bradycardia.

E. Relaxation.

The prescribed effort for training should under no circumstances exceed that of the preceding exercise test.

11. Subjects with angina pectoris should at first engage in short duration exercises with intervening rest periods until the cardiac response during exercise and recovery is known (using ECG monitoring).

12. Frequent personal contact should be especially built into any program to insure meaningful subject feedback.

13. Physical training, dietary advice, and guidance in changing patterns of daily living must be approached on a long range basis with frequent reinforcement and consideration of the subject's problems of readjustment. Promoting "fear of death" as a stimulant to motivation is *not* compatible with eventual success. Excessive claims must be avoided.

14. Regular supervised physical training is not dangerous for the coronary subject if his initial examination and his cardiac response to exercise have been accurately assessed at the outset, and if attention is paid to detecting changes during the program.

15. Unsupervised jogging as a physical training activity must be considered out of the question for unfit men over thirty years of age unless effort testing has established that the subject can tolerate this energy requirement without untoward effects.

Physical fitness cannot be strictly considered a medicine in that it is free to be used by everyone, and it is important to general health and well-being in a way similar to that of a balanced diet. On the other hand, as far as NCP and ASHD subjects are concerned, physical training must be treated as a medication in that it is only efficacious and safe as the clinical judgment which accompanies its use.

Although the value of physical fitness is widely accepted among physicians, many refuse to allow their NCP and ASHD patients to participate in physical activity programs. In our experience the main objection relates to a lack of available programs and supervision to prevent complications. In such cases this objection is quite justified. It is necessary to improve programs to meet and exceed the basic requirements of safety. Historically it would be a giant step backward to exclude the majority of our male population from physical training programs as an alternative rather than improving the efficacy, safety, and medical value of such programs.

One must at the same time acknowledge with great respect those YMCA fitness educators who have in recent years expended much effort toward obtaining adequate medical supervision of their programs. These requests have been largely unfulfilled either because an appropriate physician was not available or because of local budgetary restrictions.

The provision of adequate facilities and personnel to enhance physical fitness at all ages is one of the important challenges which faces our society.

REFERENCES

1. Eckstein, R. W.: Effect of exercise and coronary artery narrowing on collateral circulation. *Circ Res, 5*:230, 1957.
2. Hellerstein, H. K., Hirsch, E. Z., Cumler, W., Allen, L., Polster, S., and Zucker, N.: Reconditioning of the coronary patient. A preliminary report. In Likoff, W., and Moyer, J. H. (Eds.): *Coronary Heart Disease.* New York, Grune and Stratton, 1963, p. 448.
3. Sloman, G., Pitt, A., Hirsch, E. Z., and Donaldson, A.: Effect of a graded physical training programme on the physical working capacity of patients with heart disease. *Med J Aust, 1*:4, 1965.
4. Barry, A. J., Daly, I. W., Pruett, E. D. R., Steinmetz, J. R., Birkhead, N. C., and Rodahl, K.: Effects of physical training on patients who have had myocardial infarction. *Amer J Cardiol, 17*:1, 1966.
5. Kaufman, J. M., and Anslow, R. D.: Treatment of refractory angina pectoris with nitroglycerin and graded exercise. *JAMA, 196*:137, 1966.
6. Naughton, J., Shanbour, K., Armstrong, R., McCoy, J., and Lategola, M. T.: Cardiovascular responses to exercise following myocardial infarction. *Arch Intern Med, 117*:541, 1966.
7. Varnauskas, E., Bergman, H., Houk, P., and Bjorntorp, P.: Hemodynamic effects of physical training in coronary patients. *Lancet, 2*:8, 1966.
8. Hellerstein, H. K., Hornsten, T. R., Goldbarg, A. N., Burlando, A. G., Friedman, E. H., Hirsch, E. Z., and Marik, S.: The influence of active conditioning upon coronary atherosclerosis. In Brest, A. N., and Moyer, J. H. (Eds.): *Atherosclerotic Vascular Disease. A Hahnemann Symposium.* New York, Appleton-Century-Crofts, 1967, p. 115.
9. Rechnitzer, P. A., Yuhasz, M. S., Paivio, A., Pickard, H. A., and Lescoe, N.: Effect of a 24-week exercise program on normal adults and patients with previous myocardial infarction. *Brit Med J, 1*:734, 1967.

10. Wassermil, M., and Toor, M.: Effect of graded work exercise in 100 patients with ischemic heart disease: Two year follow-up. In Raab, W. (Ed.): *Prevention of Ischemic Heart Disease: Principles and Practice*. Springfield, Charles C Thomas, 1967, p. 348.

11. Zohmann, L. R., and Tobis, J. S.: Effect of exercise training on patients with angina pectoris. *Arch Physiol Med, 48*:525, 1967.

12. Bruner, D., and Meshulem, N.: Prevention of recurrent myocardial infarction by physical exercise. In Eliakim, M. (Ed.): *Proceedings of the Fourth Asian-Pacific Congress of Cardiology*. New York, Academic Press, 1969, p. 341.

13. Frick, M. H., and Katila, M.: Hemodynamic consequences of physical training after myocardial infarction. *Circulation, 37*:192, 1968.

14. Gottheiner, V.: Long-range strenuous sports training for cardiac reconditioning and rehabilitation. *Amer J Cardiol, 22*:426, 1968.

15. Kattus, A. A., Jr., Discussants: Hanafee, W. N., Longmire, W. P., Jr., MacAlpin, R. N., and Rivin, A. U.: The UCLA Interdepartmental Conference: Diagnosis, medical and surgical management of coronary insufficiency. *Ann Intern Med, 69*:115, 1968.

16. Clausen, J. P., Larsen, O. A., and Trap-Jensen, J.: Physical training in the management of coronary artery disease. *Circulation, 40*:143, 1969.

17. Goldwater, L. J., Bronstein, L. H., and Kresky, B.: *The Work Classification Unit. A Guide for its Use in the Selective Placement of Persons with Heart Disease*. American Heart Association, New York, 1951.

18. Levine, S. A., and Lown, B.: The "chair" treatment of acute coronary thrombosis. *Trans Ass Amer Physicians, 64*:316, 1951.

19. Parran, T. V., Hellerstein, H. K., Cohen, D., and Goldston, E.: Results of studies at the Work Classification Clinic of the Cleveland Area Heart Society. In Rosenbaum, F. F., and Belknap, E. L. (Eds.): *Work and the Heart*. New York, Hoeber, 1959, p. 330.

20. Rosenbaum, F. F., and Belknap, E. L. (Eds.): *Work and the Heart: Transactions of the First Wisconsin Conference on Work and the Heart*. New York, Hoeber, 1959.

21. Morris, J. N., Heady, J. A., Raffle, P. A. B., Roberts, C. G., and Parks, J. W.: Coronary heart disease and physical activity of work. *Lancet, 2*:1053, 1111, 1953.

22. Frank, C. W., Weinblatt, E., Shapiro, S., and Sager, R.: Physical inactivity as a lethal factor in myocardial infarction among men. *Circulation, 34*:1022, 1966.

23. Epstein, F.: Multiple risk factors and the prediction of coronary heart disease. *Bull NY Acad Med, 44*:916, 1968.

24. Fox, S. M., III, and Haskell, W. L.: Physical activity and the prevention of coronary heart disease. *Bull NY Acad Med, 44*:936, 1968.

25. Dawber, T. R., Moore, F. E., and Mann, G. V.: Coronary heart disease in the Framingham Study. *Amer J Public Health, 47*:4, 1957.
26. Gertler, M. M., Woodbury, M. A., Gottsch, L. G., White, P. D., and Rusk, H. A.: The candidate for coronary heart disease: Discriminating power of biochemical, hereditary and anthropometric measurements. *JAMA, 170*:149, 1959.
27. Paul, O., Lepper, M. H., Phelan, W. H., Dupertuis, G. W., MacMillan, A., McKean, H., and Park, H.: A longitudinal study of coronary heart disease. *Circulation, 28*:20, 1963.
28. Kannel, W. B., and McNamara, P. M.: The evidence for excess risk. *Minn Med, 52*:19, 1969.
29. Lown, B., Amarasingham, R., and Neuman, J.: New method for terminating cardiac arrhythmias. *JAMA, 182*:548, 1962.
30. Day, H. W.: An intensive coronary care area. *Dis Chest, 44*:423, 1963.
31. Hellerstein, H. K., and Turell, D. J.: The mode of death in coronary artery disease. An electrocardiographic and clinicopathological correlation. In Surawicz, B. (Ed.): *Sudden Cardiac Death.* New York, Grune and Stratton, 1964, p. 17.
32. Julian, D. G., Valentine, P. A., and Miller, G.: Disturbances of rate, rhythm and conduction in acute myocardial infarction. *Amer J Med, 37*:915, 1964.
33. Hellerstein, H. K.: Exercise therapy in coronary disease. *Bull NY Acad Med, 44*:1028, 1968.
34. Hellerstein, H. K., and collaborators: Bernstein, I., Burlando, A., Dupertuis, C. W., Feil, G., Friedman, E., Goldbarg, A. N., Hirsch, E. Z., Hornsten, T. R., Maistelman, H., Marik, S., Plotkin, F., Radke, J. D., Ricklin, R., Salzman, S. H., and Winkler, O.: The effects of physical activity. A community program and study among patients and normal coronary prone subjects. *Minn Med, 52*:127, 1969.
35. Kraus, H., and Raab, W.: *Hypokinetic Disease.* Springfield, Charles C Thomas, 1961.
36. Enos, W. F., Holmes, R. H., and Beyer, J.: Coronary disease among United States soldiers killed in action in Korea. *JAMA, 152*:1090, 1953.
37. Yater, W. M., Traum, A. H., Brown, W. G., Fitzgerald, R. P., Geisler, M. A., and Wilcox, B. B.: Coronary artery disease in men 18 to 39 years of age: Report of 866 cases, 450 with necropsy examination. *Amer Heart J, 36*:334, 481, 683, 1948.
38. Mattingly, T. W., Robb, G. P., and Marks, H. H.: Stress tests in the detection of coronary disease. *Postgrad Med, 24*:4, 1958.
39. Frank, C. W.: The course of coronary heart disease: Factors relating to prognosis. *Bull NY Acad Med, 44*:900, 1968.
40. Friedman, M., and Rosenman, R. H.: Association of specific overt be-

havior with blood and cardiovascular findings: Blood cholesterol level, blood clotting time, incidence of arcus senilis and clinical coronary artery disease. *JAMA, 169*:1286, 1959.

41. Friedman, E. H., and Hellerstein, H. K.: Occupational stress, law school hierarchy, and coronary artery disease in Cleveland attorneys. *Psychosom Med, 30*:72, 1968.

42. Dahlstrom, W. G., and Welsh, G. S.: *An MMPI Handbook. A Guide to Use in Clinical Practice and Research.* University of Minnesota Press, Minneapolis, 1960.

43. Sheldon, W. H., Dupertuis, C. W., and McDermott, E.: *Atlas of Men. A Guide and Handbook on Somatotyping.* New York, Harper, 1954.

44. Van Dobëln, W. A.: A simple bicycle ergometer. *J Appl Physiol, 7*:222, 1954.

45. Hellerstein, H. K., and Hornsten, T. R.: Assessing and preparing the patient for return to a meaningful and productive life. *J Rehab, 32*:48, 1966.

46. Åstrand, P. O., and Ryhming, I.: A nomogram for calculation of aerobic capacity (physical fitness) from pulse rate during submaximal work. *J Appl Physiol, 7*:218, 1954.

47. Anderson, K. L.: Measurement of maximal oxygen uptake and related respiratory and circulatory functions. Proposal to I. B. P. Handbook, Private Printing, 1967.

48. Katz, L. N., and Feinberg, H.: The relation of cardiac effort to myocardial oxygen consumption and coronary flow. *Circ Res, 6*:656, 1958.

49. Sarnoff, S. T., Braunwald, E., Welch, G. H., Case, R. B., Stainsby, W. N., and Macruz, R.: Hemodynamic determinants of oxygen consumption of the heart with special reference to the tension-time index. *Amer J Physiol, 192*:148, 1958.

50. Lester, F. M., Sheffield, L. T., and Reeves, J. T.: Electrocardiographic changes in clinically normal older men following near maximal and maximal exercise. *Circulation, 36*:5, 1967.

51. Arbaquez, R. F., Freiman, A. H., Reichel, F., and LaDue, J. S.: The precordial electrocardiogram during exercise. *Circulation, 22*:1060, 1960.

52. Salzman, S. H., Hellerstein, H. K., Radke, J. D., Maistelman, H. M., and Ricklin, R.: Quantitative effects of physical conditioning on the exercise electrocardiogram of middle-aged subjects with arteriosclerotic heart disease. In Blackburn, H. (Ed.): *Measurement in Exercise Electrocardiography.* Springfield, Charles C Thomas, 1969, p. 388.

53. Hellerstein, H. K., Friedman, E. H., Brdar, P. J., Weiss, M., Dupertuis, C. W., Turell, D. J., and Rumbaugh, D.: A comparison of the

personality of adult subjects with rheumatic heart disease and with arteriosclerotic heart disease. An ecologic approach to behavioral patterns. Presented at the Meeting of Scientific Council on Rehabilitation of the International Society of Cardiology, Hohenried, Germany, June 18, 1969. (In press).

54. Hirsch, E. Z.: The effects of digoxin on the electrocardiogram after strenuous exercise in normal men. *Amer Heart J, 70*:196, 1965.

55. Blackburn, H.: The exercise electrocardiogram. Technological procedural and conceptual developments. In Blackburn, H. (Ed.): *Measurement in Exercise Electrocardiography.* Charles C Thomas, Springfield, 1969, p. 220.

56. Goodman, D. S., and Noble, R. P.: Turnover of plasma cholesterol in man. *J Clin Invest, 47*:231, 1968.

57. Fredrickson, D. S., Levy, R. I., and Lees, R. S.: Fat transport in lipoproteins—an integrated approach to mechanisms and disorders. *New Eng J Med, 276*:148, 1967.

58. Feil, H.: *Coronary Heart Disease. A Personal Clinical Study.* Springfield, Charles C Thomas, 1964.

59. Blackburn, H.: The current developments in North America. Presented at the Second International Symposium on Atherosclerosis, Chicago, November 2-5, 1969. (In press).

60. Hellerstein, H. K.: Relation of exercise to acute myocardial infarction. *Circulation, 40 (supp. IV)*:124, 1969.

61. Weinberg, S., and Helpern, M.: Circumstances related to sudden, unexpected death in coronary heart disease. In Rosenbaum, F. F., and Belknap, E. L. (Eds.).: *Work and the Heart,* Hoeber, New York, 1959, p. 288.

62. Schettler, G.: Keynote address. Presented at the Second International Symposium on Atherosclerosis, Chicago, November 2-5, 1969. (In press).

63. Harris, A. S., Bisteni, A., Russell, R. A., Brigham, I. C., and Firestone, J. E.: Excitatory factors in ventricular tachycardia resulting from myocardial ischemia. Potassium a major excitant. *Science, 119*:200, 1954.

64. Parker, J. O., West, R. O., Case, R. B., and Chiong, M. A.: Temporal relationships of myocardial lactate metabolism, left ventricular function, and S-T segment depression during angina precipitated by exercise. *Circulation, 40*:97, 1969.

65. Parker, J. O., Chiong, M. A., West, R. O., and Case, R. B.: Sequential alterations in myocardial lactate metabolism and left ventricular function during angina induced by atrial pacing. *Circulation, 40*:113, 1969.

66. Hanson, J. S., Tabakin, B. S., Levy, A. M., and Nedde, W.: Long-term

physical training and cardiovascular dynamics in middle-aged men. *Circulation, 38*:783, 1968.

67. Epstein, S. E., Robinson, B. F., Kahler, R. L., and Braunwald, E.: Effects of beta-adrenergic blockade on the cardiac response to maximal and submaximal exercise in man. *J Clin Invest, 44*:1745, 1965.

68. Gianelly, R. E., Treister, B. L., and Harrison, D. C.: The effect of propranolol on exercise-induced ischemic S-T segment depression. *Amer J Cardiol, 24*:161, 1969.

69. Goldbarg, A. N., Moran, J. F., Butterfield, T. K., Nemickas, R., and Bermudez, G. A.: Therapy of angina pectoris with propranolol and long-acting nitrates. *Circulation, 40*:847, 1969.

70. Kireilis, R. W., and Cureton, T. K.: The relationships of external fat to physical education activities and fitness tests. *Res Quart, 18*:123, 1947.

71. Mann, G. V., and White H. S.: Influence of stress on plasma cholesterol levels. *Metabolism, 2*:47, 1953.

72. Mann, G. V., Teel, K., Hayes, O., McHailey, H., and Bruno, D.: Exercise in the disposition of dietary calories. *New Eng J Med, 253*:439, 1955.

73. Keys, A., Anderson, J. T., and Mickelson, O.: Serum cholesterol in men in basal and non-basal states. *Science, 123*:29, 1956.

74. Keys, A., Anderson, J. T., Aresu, M., Biörck, G., Brock, J. F., Bronte-Stewart, B., Fidanza, F., Keys, M. H., Malmros, H., Poppi, A., Posteli, T., Swahn, B., and del Vecchio, A.: Physical activity and the diet in populations differing in serum cholesterol. *J Clin Invest, 35*:1173, 1956.

75. Kobernick, S. D., Niwayama, G., and Zuchlewski, A. C.: Cholesterol effects reduced by exercise. *Proc Soc Exp Biol Med, 96*:623, 1957.

76. Taylor, H. L., Anderson, J. T., and Keys, A.: Effect on serum lipids of 1,300 calories of daily walking. *Fed Proc, 16*:128, 1957.

77. Pohndorf, R. H.: Cholesterol studies: A review. *Res Quart, 29*:180, 1958.

78. Gordon, E. S.: The effect of exercise on lipid metabolism. In *Colloquium on the Scientific Aspects of Exercise and Fitness.* University of Illinois Press, Urbana, 1959, p. 96.

79. Johnson, T., Wong, H., Shim, R., Liu, B., and Hall, A.: The influence of exercise on serum cholesterol, phospholipids and electrophoretic serum protein patterns in college swimmers. *Fed Proc, 18*:77, 1959.

80. Montoye, H. J., VanHuss, W. D., Brewer, W. D., Jones, E. M., Ohlson, M. A., Mahoney, E., and Olson, H.: The effects of exercise on blood cholesterol in middle-aged men. *Amer J Clin Nutr, 7*:139, 1959.

81. Brumbach, W. B.: Changes in the serum cholesterol levels of male college students who participated in a special physical exercise program. *Res Quart, 32*:147, 1961.

82. Golding, L.: The effects of physical training upon total serum cholesterol levels. *Res Quart, 32*:499, 1961.

83. Rochelle, R.: Blood plasma cholesterol changes during a physical training program. *Res Quart, 32*:538, 1961.

84. Bruner, D., Loebl, K., and Altman, S.: Influence of manual labor on lipid values and their relation to the incidence of coronary artery disease. *Circulation, 26 (suppl. 2)*: 693, 1962.

85. Holloszy, J. O., Skinner, J. S., Toro, G., and Cureton, T. K.: Effects of a six month program on endurance exercise on the serum lipids of middle-aged men. *Amer J Cardiol, 14*:753, 1964.

86. Campbell, D. E.: Influence of several physical activities on serum cholesterol concentrations in young men. *J Lipid Res, 6*:478, 1965.

87. Naughton, J., and McCoy, J. F.: Observations on the relationships of physical activity to the serum cholesterol concentration of healthy men and cardiac patients. *J Chronic Dis, 19*:727, 1966.

88. Shane, S. R.: Relation between serum lipids and physical conditioning. *Amer J Cardiol, 18*:540, 1966.

89. Goode, R., Firstbrook, J., and Shephard, R.: Effects of exercise and a cholesterol free diet on human serum lipids. *Canad J Physiol Pharmacol, 44*:575, 1966.

90. Campbell, D. E.: Influence of diet and physical activity on blood serum cholesterol of young adult males. *Amer J Clin Nutr, 18*:79, 1966.

91. Mann, G. V., Garret, H. L., Farhi, A., Murray, H., Billings, F. T., with the assistance of: Schute, E., and Schwarten, S. E.: Exercise to prevent coronary heart diseases. An experimental study of the effects of training on risk factors for coronary disease in man. *Amer J Med, 46*:12, 1969.

92. Campbell, D. E.: Effect of controlled running on serum cholesterol of young adult males of varying morphological constitutions. *Res Quart, 39*:47, 1967.

93. Berkson, D. M., Whipple, I. T., Sime, W. E., Lerner, H., Berstein, I., MacIntyre, W., and Stamler, J.: Experience with a long term supervised ergometric exercise program for middle-aged sedentary American men. *Circulation, 36 (suppl. 2)*: 67, 1967.

94. Skinner, J. S., Holloszy, J. O., and Cureton, T. K.: Effects of a program of endurance exercises on physical work capacity and anthropometric measurements of 15 middle-aged men. *Amer J Cardiol, 14*:747, 1964.

95. Carlson, L. A.: Lipid metabolism and muscular work. *Fed Proc, 26*:1755, 1967.

96. Farquhar, J. W., Gross, R. C., Wagner, R. M., and Reaven, G. M.: Validation of an incompletely coupled two compartment non-recycling catenary model for turnover of liver and plasma tryglyceride in man. *J Lipid Res, 6*:119, 1965.

97. Radke, J. D., Hellerstein, H. K., Miller, M., and Pearson, O. H.: In-

fluence of physical training on the glucose tolerance test, immuno-reactive insulin, and growth hormone. In preparation.

98. Davidson, P. C., Shane, S. R., and Albrink, M. J.: Decreased glucose tolerance following a physical conditioning program. *Circulation, 34 (suppl. 3)*:7, 1966.

99. Moses, C. (Medical Director of the American Heart Association): Personal communication.

100. Johnson, H. J.: Warning to joggers from a leading physician. *U. S. News and World Report, 47*:74, 1969.

101. Pyfer, H. R., and Doane, B. L.: Cardiac arrest during exercise training. *JAMA, 210*:101, 1969.

102. Bruce, R. A., Hornsten, T. R., and Blackmon, J. R.: Myocardial infarction after normal responses to maximal exercise. *Circulation, 38*:552, 1968.

103. Saltin, B., Blumquist, G., Mitchell, J. H., Johnson, R. L. Jr., Wildenthal, K., and Chapman, C. B.: Response to exercise after bed rest and after training. American Heart Association Monograph Number 23, New York, 1968.

104. Gruen, J. J.: Presentation at the Second International Symposium on Atherosclerosis, Chicago, November 2-5, 1969. (In press).

105. Simonov, P. V.: Studies of emotional behavior of humans and animals by Soviet physiologists. *Ann NY Acad Sci, 159*:1112, 1969.

APPENDIX I

Training Classification Categories

T1 *Trained 1*. Negative history, physical examination, electrocardiogram, and normal "trained" heart rate and blood pressure response to exercise.

T2 *Trained 2*. Same as 1 except more than 10 percent, less than 20 percent overweight.

U1 *Untrained Normal*. Same as T1 except "untrained" response to exercise.

U2 *Untrained Normal (overweight)*. Same as U1 except more than 10 percent and less than 20 percent overweight.

L1 *Limited 1*. Normal resting electrocardiogram, "untrained" heart rate and blood pressure response to exercise, and any one of the following:

(1) More than 20 percent and less than 25 percent overweight.

(2) History of questionably significant chest pain.

(3) Diastolic hypertension (less than 110 mm) at rest, reduced to 95 mm or less with medication.

(4) Grossly abnormal unexplained vital capacity.

(5) Poor vasomotor response to bike test (drop in blood pressure on increasing work loads).

(6) Family history of coronary artery disease and age more than fifty years old.

(7) Family history of coronary artery disease and
a) smokes more than one pack of cigarettes per day or
b) markedly high saturated fat source in diet.

L2 *Limited 2*. Normal "untrained" response to exercise tests and any one of the following:

(1) Diastolic blood pressure more than 110 mm reduced to 95 mm or less with medication.

(2) History and physical examination of compensated mitral valvular disease.

(3) Significantly abnormal physical examination of heart or lungs.

(4) Significant family history of coronary artery disease and arcus or xanthomata.

(5) Abnormal flack test and any other significant finding to indicate possible cardiac disease.

(6) Resting electrocardiogram evidence of ventricular hypertrophy, aberrant A-V, I-V conduction and left bundle branch block (isolated right bundle branch block excluded).

S1 *Supervised 1.* Any one of the following:

(1) Diastolic blood pressure more than 110 mm, reduced to 95 mm or less with medication, plus ECG evidence of left ventricular hypertrophy with normal untrained response to exercise tests while taking medication.

(2) History or ECG evidence of angina or myocardial infarction with negative ECG response at effort requiring a heart rate of 150 beats per minute.

(3) ST abnormality which appears progressively during exercise tests.

(4) Ventricular or atrial arrhythmias (except premature atrial beats) which appear or increase on exercise tests with no history nor symptoms suggesting coronary artery disease.

S2 *Supervised 2.* Any one of the following:

(1) Cardiac symptoms with abnormal ECG response to exercise test.

(2) ECG evidence of myocardial infarction with abnormal ECG response to exercise tests.

Excluded

(1) More than 25 percent overweight.

(2) Evidence of changing myocardial process.

(3) Aortic or significant pulmonary stenosis or aortic insufficiency with or without symptoms.

(4) Mitral valvular disease with symptoms at rest.

(5) Congestive heart failure.

Any cardiopulmonary diseases other than those listed above are placed according to clinical judgment.

APPENDIX II

Monthly Exercise Prescription
Jewish Community Center
of Cleveland

_____

No. & Group

NAME_____

ADDRESS_____
(If Changed)

TELEPHONE (Office)_____ (Home)_____

ACTIVITY RECORD FROM_____ to_____

_____Month of Training

This is your physical fitness training program which you are asked to follow at least *three times a week*. Record all your activities as prescribed on the calendar as indicated. If for any reason you deviate from your prescription, describe what happended (date, time and activity) under "Remarks". Use other side if necessary. Return this record sheet at the end of the month and secure a new one from the Physical Education office. *This record will become part of your personal physical fitness portfolio.*

CONDITIONING CLASS (30 Minutes)
Record your attendance by "X-ing" calendar below.

<table>
<tr><td></td><td colspan="3">Regular Count</td><td></td><td></td><td></td><td></td><td></td><td></td><td></td></tr>
<tr><td></td><td>24</td><td>36</td><td>48</td><td></td><td></td><td></td><td></td><td></td><td></td><td></td></tr>
<tr><td>Week</td><td colspan="3">Your Count</td><td>SUN</td><td>MON</td><td>TUE</td><td>WED</td><td>THUR</td><td>FRI</td><td>SAT</td></tr>
<tr><td>1</td><td></td><td></td><td></td><td></td><td></td><td></td><td></td><td></td><td></td><td></td></tr>
<tr><td>2</td><td></td><td></td><td></td><td></td><td></td><td></td><td></td><td></td><td></td><td></td></tr>
<tr><td>3</td><td></td><td></td><td></td><td></td><td></td><td></td><td></td><td></td><td></td><td></td></tr>
<tr><td>4</td><td></td><td></td><td></td><td></td><td></td><td></td><td></td><td></td><td></td><td></td></tr>
<tr><td>5</td><td></td><td></td><td></td><td></td><td></td><td></td><td></td><td></td><td></td><td></td></tr>
</table>

ADDITIONAL INSTRUCTIONS:

1. Do you have chest discomfort during or after exercises?
2. Have you been unusually fatigued?
3. Has there been any change in your ability to do the exercises?

ENDURANCE ACTIVITY   INTERVAL RUNNING
(Record Total Number of Laps RUN each time in.)
  If on a walking program, record minutes
  and number of laps completed.

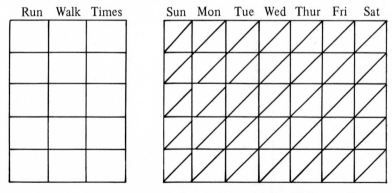

Run	Walk	Times		Sun	Mon	Tue	Wed	Thur	Fri	Sat

ALWAYS WALK AT LEAST *3* LAPS BRISKLY *BEFORE* AND
AT *COMPLETION* OF RUNNING.

  Advance to next week's level of activity only
  if you exercised at least 3 times during
  previous week.
REMARKS:

RECREATION ACTIVITY (15 Minutes)
Mark days with letter identifying activity.
For outside activities more than 15 minutes
indicate sport and date below.

Exercise Room

A Rowing Machine
B Bicycle
C Treadmill
D Punching Bag
E Wall Pulley

Gym

F Volleyball
G Basketball
H Badminton

Pool

I Recreation
J Instruction
K Distance

Courts

L Handball
M Paddleball
N Squash

	Sun	Mon	Tue	Wed	Thur	Fri	Sat

OUTSIDE
ACTIVITY:

Glossary of Terms Supplemental
to Definitions in the Text

Work Load 150
(WL$_{150}$)
—work performance or work tolerance as an index of fitness, measured as the power (kg meters per min) at which a subject's heart rate (HR) reaches or would be expected to reach 150 beats per minute.

"Serum enzymes"
—enzymes such as Creatine Phosphokinase and S.G.O.T. which are released into the circulation from myocardial muscle when cell death takes place.

Intercoronary
Anastomoses
—so-called collateral circulation which consists of small arterial channels which develop, circumventing coronary artery obstructive lesions, to enhance blood supply to hypoxic areas of the myocardium.

Cardiac Output (CO)
—minute output of blood from the heart in liters per minute.

Cardiac Index (CI)
—CO per square meter body surface area = (CO/M^2 B.S.A.) in liters per minute.

Stroke Volume (SV)
—amount of blood ejected with each beat in milliliters per beat.

Stroke Index (SI)
—SV/M^2 B.S.A. in milliliters.

Systolic Ejection
Period (SEP)
—time during which blood is ejected during systole.

Ejection Time
Index (ETI)
—SEP corrected for heart rate = SEP + .0016 HR in seconds.

Left Ventricular
Mean Systolic
Pressure (LVSPm)
—mean pressure during SEP.

Left Ventricular
End Diastolic
Pressure (LVED)   —self explanatory.

Tension Time   —an important determinant and approxi-
Index (TTI)   mate equivalent of myocardial oxygen con-
    sumption $= (\text{LVSPm} \times \text{HR} \times \text{SEP})$.

Left Ventricular   —index of left ventricular mechanical work
Minute Work Index   per minute $= \dfrac{(\text{LVSPm} - \text{LVED}) \times \text{CI} \times 1.36}{100}$ kg meters/min/M^2
(LVMWI)

Left Ventricular   —index of left ventricular mechanical work
Stroke Work Index   per stroke $= \dfrac{(\text{LVSPm} - \text{LVED}) \times \text{SI} \times 1.36}{100}$ kg meters/beat/M^2
(LVSWI)

Mean Systolic Ejection—index of mean rate of ejection from the left
Rate Index (MSERI)   ventricle during systole $= \dfrac{\text{SI}}{\text{SEP}}$ ml/sec/beat

Left Ventricular   —volume of blood contained by left ventricle
Volume (LVV)   (usually at end diastole).

Ejection Fraction   —$\dfrac{\text{LV end diastolic volume} - \text{LV end systolic volume}}{\text{LV end diastolic volume}}$
(EF)   expressed as a percentage.

Left Ventricular   —$\dfrac{\text{LVMWI}}{\text{TTI}} \times 1000$
Efficiency Index
(LVEI)

Chapter 9

DISABLING COMPLICATIONS OF PHYSICAL EXERCISE TRAINING IN MIDDLE - AGE, CORONARY - PRONE AMERICAN MEN

BURT B. HAMRELL.* HENRY BLACKBURN,
AND HENRY L. TAYLOR

PHYSICAL exercise is a new and unproven medical therapeutic approach in coronary heart disease. When exercise is advised as a possible preventive against coronary heart disease, disabling complications of exercise must be regarded more seriously than injuries from physical exertion undertaken as a sport. Proper evaluation of exercise as a medical regimen depends on cooperative efforts between physicians and physical educators. Documentation of changes in cardiovascular fitness and complications of exercise will allow the physical education-physician team to make a balanced assessment of an exercise program and institute appropriate immediate alterations. Systematic review of such data will lead to improvement of future programs.

Previous chapters presented the mechanisms of the physiologic effects of physical exercise, modes of administration of exercise, and the selection of suitable subjects for activity programs. Therapeutic regimens may seem promising initially because side effects and complications receive little attention due to insufficient experience. Some complications require months or years to become apparent. This is the classical therapeutic "pendulum." With current interest in unsupervised exercise programs proposed to prolong life and prevent heart attacks, the "pendulum" is somewhere in an enthusiastic swing to the left. This symposium and other recent meetings (1)

---

* The research described here was done during Dr. Hamrell's tenure as a Public Health Service Officer assigned to the Laboratory of Physiological Hygiene by the Heart Disease and Stroke Control Program. He is currently in the Departments of Physiology and Medicine, College of Medicine, University of Vermont, Burlington, Vermont.

suggest that the pendulum has begun to swing back toward the middle. Long-term study and accumulated experience eventually lead to a balanced assessment of the efficacy of a treatment in relation to the dangers of administration. This discussion is an initial attempt at such an assessment.

BACKGROUND OF THE COLLABORATIVE EXERCISE PROGRAMS

In the 1960's a working group assembled by Dr. Samuel M. Fox, III of the Public Health Service's Heart Disease and Stroke Control Program decided on the basis of available data to initiate pilot studies to define the problems of mounting a definitive physical exercise intervention study. The purpose of a definitive study would be to evaluate whether an increase in physical activity level in a random sample of the population would result in a subsequent decrease in the incidence of coronary heart disease as compared with a matched control group from the same sample. The requirements of sample size and staffing led to the decision to use "coronary-prone" middlea-fe men. Pilot studies were organized at the University of Wisconsin directed by Dr. Bruno Balke, at Pennsylvania State University directed by Dr. Elsworth Buskirk and at the University of Minnesota directed by Dr. Henry Taylor. The following comments refer to the latter study.

Recruitment

In Minneapolis, from 13,500 households telephoned, close to 11,000 were contacted by a trained, experienced interviewer after each household received an introductory letter. The interviewer determined whether a man, aged forty-five through fifty-four years, currently lived at that household; 1,528 age-eligible men were found. Of these, 1,331 completed the telephone interview and were invited to a brief health examination at a local school.

Risk Examination

Of those invited, 979 age-eligible men kept their appointment to the health examination where coronary heart disease risk factor data were gathered including:

(1) Smoking habit history

(2) Physical activity habit history

(3) Serum cholesterol level

(4) Sitting blood pressure level

(5) Triceps and subscapular skinfold thickness

(6) Height and weight

Risk Classification

From the 979 men examined, 493 were selected as "coronary-prone" based primarily on an elevated serum cholesterol level, and partly on an elevated blood pressure level and/or a history of excessive cigarette smoking.

All men designated "coronary-prone" were invited to one of several recruitment meetings; 348 attended and 213 volunteered for the study. They volunteered with the understanding that later random division of the volunteer group would assign one half of the men to three one-hour supervised exercise sessions per week and the other half to a control group.

Medical Examination

The 177 volunteers (there were 36 "no-shows") were examined medically, and of the men examined 42 were excluded for medical factors similar to those discussed by Dr. W. Kannel in an earlier chapter, including conditions likely to prevent safe and regular adherence to the program, or likely to require considerable outside medical direction. Those who passed the medical examination entered a one-month testing and "faint-of-heart" period. During that period ten men dropped out because of lack of interest. A detailed testing program eliminated another ten men for medical reasons including abnormal responses to motor-driven treadmill work, and left 115 men. These successfully completed the period, including testing with a continuous 3 mph treadmill walk with progressive grade increments of 2.5 percent each two minutes, to a work load which elicited a heart rate of 150 beats/minute, approximately 70 percent of the estimated maximal heart rate for this age group.

Exercise Program

The fifty-seven men randomly assigned to the exercise group entered into a gradually progressive exercise program beginning with low energy level isotonic calisthenics and noncontact, noncompetitive games supervised by staff members and graduate students of the University of Minnesota Physical Education Department. The calisthenics were designed to stretch and strengthen lower extremity, back and abdominal muscles, tendons and ligaments important in jogging.

During the second month of the program, jogging was instituted. Each man was assigned an individualized jogging prescription based on the initial treadmill stress testing results and expressed in terms of a sequence of jogging and walking laps around the perimeter of the gymnasium floor. The initial prescriptions were conservative in order to ensure that the men did not exceed the heart rate attained during treadmill work, i.e. 150 beats per minute.

The jogging program was monitored by the men who palpated and counted their own carotid pulse immediately upon completion of a full prescription. These observations were corroborated by the supervising physical educator and with radio-telemetric monitoring of heart rate and electrocardiogram (no clinical episodes of hypotension occurred because of carotid sinus pressure). The men exercised up to but not beyond the 150 beat/minute heart rate limit reached during the treadmill test. During the first six months of the program the jogging prescriptions were increased by several small increments to approach this limit; after the first six months the prescriptions were advanced as rapidly as possible while staying within the 150 beat/minute limit.

The physiologic effects of the exercise program were measured in part with the 3 mph continuous treadmill test described above. The work load was observed at which each man's heart rate reached 140 beats/minute (the grade was increased 2.5% each 2 min) during the November, 1966 test. The heart rate was noted at that workload during the same test regimen in June 1967 (after 6 mos of exercise) and February 1968 (after 14 mos of exercise); the differences from the November, 1966 value were computed. The men in the exercise group were classed into quartiles of the distribution of total miles jogged over the same time periods. Figure 9-1 demonstrates the decrease in heart rate response to a fixed external workload according to the number of miles jogged. The relationship between these variables is obvious and persists throughout fourteen months of exercise. The similarity is evident between the heart rate change in the control group and that in men who jogged the least. Thus, a degree of cardiovascular conditioning was attained and as a function of the extent of participation in the pilot study at Minneapolis. Although not completely analyzed, similar results were noted at Pennsylvania State University and the University of Wisconsin.

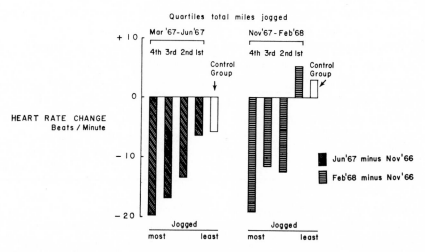

Figure 9-1. Progressive treadmill test. Group mean individual differences in heart rate response at six and fifteen months to workload in the November, 1966 baseline test that elicited a heart rate of 140 beats per minute.

Medical Complications of Exercise

In the following discussion descriptions of anatomy and pathophysiology are included to assist readers not familiar with the medical aspects of injuries related to physical exercise.

Ocular

During the initial six-week period of low-level calisthenics, a fifty-three-year-old participant was struck on the side of the head by a basketball and developed over a period of hours a progressive decrease in vision of the eye on that side. Prompt medical and surgical therapy for retinal detachment resulted in complete restitution of visual acuity. There was no prior history of visual problems other than surgically treated cataracts.

Retinal separation occurs more commonly in older age and in men (2, 3). Some consider it as one of the complications of cataract extraction (4, 5). Frequently, the symptoms are associated with a recent traumatic episode, but usually underlying retinal abnormalities are present which predispose to retinal tears and separation from the pigmented choroidal tissue.

Individuals with a past history of retinal detachment are probably poor candidates for an exercise program because of the risk of recurrent detachment and the likelihood of predisposing conditions of the other eye (5). A carefully supervised exercise regimen utilizing stationary bicycle work might be tried in cooperation with, and under the surveillance of, an ophthalomologist. Individuals who have had cataract extractions possibly have an excess risk of subsequent retinal detachment (3, 5) and should be included only in specially supervised programs.

Lower Extremity

After the first two weeks of mild jogging, a forty-nine-year-old participant complained of knee pain accompanied by swelling and tenderness. Evaluation by an orthopedic surgeon revealed a fractured articular cartilage with "joint mice," and he was advised by his physician to withdraw from the program. This subject later recalled having knee pain when he participated in contact sports as a youth. His sedentary existence as an adult may explain the lack of symptoms prior to his involvement in the exercise program.

Foreign bodies in the joint space, so-called joint mice, are secondary to fracture and detachment of portions of the menisci. The medial and lateral menisci of the knee are the fibrocartilaginous structures overlying the articular surfaces of the tibia. Damage to them is relatively unusual in other than contact sports where rotational strain or torsion can occur on a flexed, weight-bearing knee. The medial

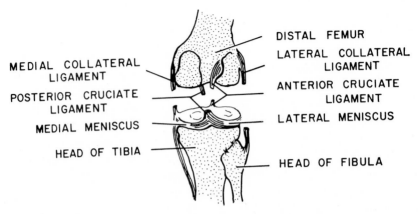

MEDIAL COLLATERAL
LIGAMENT

POSTERIOR CRUCIATE
LIGAMENT

MEDIAL MENISCUS

HEAD OF TIBIA

DISTAL FEMUR

LATERAL COLLATERAL
LIGAMENT

ANTERIOR CRUCIATE
LIGAMENT

LATERAL MENISCUS

HEAD OF FIBULA

Figure 9-2. This diagram of the posterior aspect of the knee joint illustrates the firm attachment of the medial meniscus to surrounding supportive structures.

meniscus is more commonly involved since it is more firmly fixed to surrounding ligaments than the lateral meniscus (Fig. 9-2) (6). Pain, often localized to the involved side, and limitation of motion, sometimes with locking of the joint, are the primary manifestations. A small effusion may appear, and there is often tenderness along the margin of the tibial condyle, i.e. the upper edge of the tibia. Occasionally the meniscus can be felt moving in and out, as the knee is gently flexed and extended. Treatment consists of surgical removal of the detached portion or the entire fractured meniscus.

Other causes of acute limitation of motion of the knee also require surgery, such as chondromalacia (deterioration of joint cartilage because of unknown causes but possibly related to the chronic trauma of weight-bearing exercise), and fractured articular cartilage. The definitive diagnosis is sometimes made only when the knee joint is operated on. Delay in therapy for persistent decrease in knee function may lead to quadriceps muscle wasting and joint deterioration (8).

Muscle-Tendon Rupture

One moderately obese man consistently complained of muscle stiffness and aching, particularly of the entire lower extremities. He was stiff at rest and could not seem to work out the "kinks." His jogging prescription remained low and symptom-limited during the initial four or five months of the program; then during a volleyball game he experienced severe searing left midcalf pain as he leaped vertically to hit the ball over the net. He was unable to bear weight or walk for several minutes, after which the pain changed to a dull ache, but remained well localized over the midcalf. During the next several days local calf swelling and a large hematoma appeared; a firm area was palpable at the tender site. Some suggest that this syndrome is the result of rupture of the plantaris longus, a small muscle arising from the lower lateral edge of the femur and inserting via a long thin tendon into the posterior part of the calcaneous. It lies deep to the gastrocnemius and soleus muscles. Others suggest these symptoms and signs result from rupture of fibers of the belly of the gastrocnemius. Treatment is the same regardless of the muscle involved:

(1) cold packs with pressure over the painful area for twenty-four hours

(2) no weight bearing for twenty-four hours

(3) begin local heat after the second day

Complications are unlikely, but if enough muscle is torn, functional loss will result; a persistent serum-containing pseudocyst may form from a large hematoma; slight permanent disability may result if a large hematoma calcifies and forms an island of cancellous bone, i.e. localized myositis ossificans (7). All of these complications require surgical therapy.

Exercise rehabilitation was attempted in this man, but generalized muscle stiffness persisted and culminated in withdrawal from the program.

Another case of calf muscle tear occurred in a well-conditioned man after nine months of regular exercise, when he jumped vertically during a volleyball match. This man's symptoms were less severe, and he was gradually returned to full participation. These complications suggest that exercises or games involving leaping should be avoided or delayed until after the first year of any program involving previously sedentary middle-age men.

Claudication

A fifty-year-old office worker, with diabetes of adult-onset type, responded negatively to a standardized leg-pain questionnaire (9), but noted calf "stiffness" at high work loads of the initial treadmill tests and during jogging. As the program progressed, his level of cardiovascular conditioning increased. Higher grades and longer periods on the treadmill, and more jogging laps in the program were necessary to elicit a heart rate of 150 beats per minute. At these higher workloads clear-cut symptoms of intermittent claudication appeared. He continued enthusiastic participation in the program within the limits of his leg symptoms for the full eighteen-month period. This case history is a clear example of subclinical disease brought to the surface by chronic exercise stress. Although no cause-effect relationship of arterial insufficiency with the higher workloads is implied, its appearance is reported as a "complication" to the exercise program.

Phlebitis

One man presented with a history of unilateral chronic deep and superficial venous insufficiency secondary to thrombotic episodes several years earlier. He was accepted into the study after successful completion of initial treadmill testing, the rationale being that a gradually progressive exercise regimen might decrease deep venous insufficiency by improving the muscle pumping action of the lower extremities. After a few weeks of minimal jogging an episode of superficial and deep phlebitis occurred accompanied by increased edema. His doctor advised him to discontinue the program. Whether exercise precipitated the phlebitic episode is unresolved, but careful observation is required in exercising individuals with this problem.

Other Musculoskeletal Injuries

Upper extremity problems were rare, mild, and related to specific traumatic episodes. However, other lower extremity knee and ankle problems were common and experienced intermittently to some degree by all the men throughout the program. Mild to moderate swelling and discomfort in the knee the morning after exercise may be a result of capsular sprain, and it was treated with rest and gradual resumption of exercise when the subject became symptom-free. None of the men developed joint instability and hematoma formation that would have signified underlying ligamentous tears.

The development of "shin splints" or shin soreness has been a problem in jogging programs. "Shin splints" is an ill-defined term including several diagnostic entities that involve tearing or edema with resultant ischemia of muscular attachments in the anterior and/or posterior compartments of the lower leg. Such damage is manifest by aching and tenderness of the involved areas. Several of the men experienced mild anterior lower leg discomfort, but the slowly progressive jogging regimen largely forestalled this problem.

Ankle joint swelling presumably due to capsular sprain was common, and tended to occur early in the program. Several men had intermittent ankle soreness and/or swelling throughout the program. Treatment consisted of rest and cold compresses for twenty-four hours. High top tennis shoes were considered essential for adequate ankle support.

Back Injury

One man developed a herniated lumbar disc after efforts to push the car of a lady in distress in a Minneapolis snowstorm while on the way to an exercise session. This occurred during the second month of the program, and he had not exercised for two days. This musculoskeletal event was not related to the prescribed exercise. Nevertheless, our program avoided calisthenics requiring rapid torso twisting or back flexion because of concern for this complication.

Symptom Survey

After approximately nine months of the exercise program, the entire study cohort completed a self-administered questionnaire about discomfort and swelling in the upper and lower extremities and back. Figure 9-3 illustrates the results in a bar graph. Knee and ankle discomfort and leg stiffness were more common in the exercise group, and those with joint complaints in the exercise group had associated swelling more often than did the control group. The control group had a proportionally greater experience with back discomfort; how-

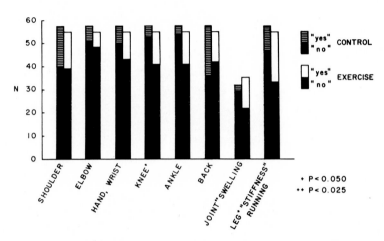

Figure 9-3. Medical interim history. The differences between the treatment and control group for knee discomfort, ankle swelling, and leg "stiffness" reached statistical significance.

ever, this difference from the exercise group was not statistically significant.

Conclusions

These phenomena are considered to be complications of exercise in previously sedentary, middle-aged, coronary-prone men selected from a stratified random sample of their community. These occurred despite a slowly progressive exercise regimen with carefully tailored prescriptions, and our comments refer specifically to the type of exercise and games used. One may avoid some of these problems by having a choice of several types of exercise, such as cycling and swimming, instead of jogging available at the outset and during the course of a training program, and by careful selection of games and recreational activities. However, regardless of the type of exercise, any definitive intervention study of the effect of an increase in physical exercise on the subsequent development of coronary heart disease must include consideration of whether the dose of physical activity has an acceptable immediate and long-term morbidity. In the meandevelop techniques for anticipating, avoiding, and managing them.

time, exercise programs offered for their potential protective effect against coronary heart disease must be undertaken with careful medical surveillance: to document and report complications and to

ACKNOWLEDGMENTS

The authors wish to express their indebtedness to Dr. John F. Alexander and other participating members of the Men's Physical Education Department of the University of Minnesota, in particular Mr. Robert Soenstrom.

Dr. E. Stanton Fetcher of the University of Minnesota's Laboratory of Physiological Hygiene was responsible for many of the administrative aspects of this study.

The work reported here was aided by a contract between the Regents of the University of Minnesota and the National Center for Chronic Disease Control (PH108-66-123) and grants from the National Center for Chronic Disease Control to H. L. Taylor for continuing support of the pilot study (CDOO333) and for support of the planning committee (CDOO118) and from the National Heart Institute to Dr. R. B. Howard for the Cardiovascular Clinical Research Program.

REFERENCES

1. Myrtle Beach Conference. Report of Proceedings on Exercise and Health at Myrtle Beach, South Carolina, May 1969. (To be published as a special issue of the South Carolina Medical Journal.)
2. Adler, F. H.: *Textbook of Ophthalmology.* Philadelphia, W. B. Saunders, 1962, pp. 394-398.
3. Schepens, C. L., and Marden, S.: Data on the Natural History of Retinal Detachment. *Arch Ophthal,* 66:631, 1961.
4. Adler, F. H.: *Textbook of Ophthalmology.* Philadelphia, W. B. Saunders, 1962, p. 507.
5. Adams, S. T.: Annual review: Retina and optic nerve. *Arch Ophthal,* 69:642, 1963.
6. O'Donoghue, D. H.: *Treatment of Injuries to Athletes.* Philadelphia, W. B. Saunders, 1962, pp. 494-502.
7. Williams, J. G. (Ed.): *Sports Medicine.* Baltimore, Williams and Wilkins, 1962, pp. 279-284.
8. Williams, J. G. (Ed.): *Sports Medicine.* Baltimore, Williams and Wilkins, 1962, pp. 79-97.
9. Rose, G. A., and Blackburn, H.: *Cardiovascular Survey Methods.* Geneva, World Health Organization, 1968, pp. 173-174.

Chapter 10

LETHAL COMPLICATIONS OF EXERCISE*

BERNARD LOWN AND BERNARD D. KOSOWSKY

At present there is no convincing evidence that regular physical activity or exercise lessens the incidence of atherosclerotic heart disease or of its major complications such as myocardial infarction and sudden death (1). Nevertheless, cumulating data suggests that exercise provides a salutory effect for patients with ischemic heart disease (2). Certainly it facilitates rehabilitation and restoration of functional capacity in those recovering from acute myocardial infarction. Exercise conditioning diminishes the incidence of angina pectoris, and even if illusory, provides an enhanced physical and psychological sense of well-being. Exercise conditioning programs are being widely recommended by physicians for patients with established coronary heart disease. Exercise is being increasingly undertaken by middle aged males, many of whom, no doubt, have significant but undiagnosed impairment of the coronary circulation. It is therefore relevant to determine the type of hazards which the cardiac patient may face while exercising. In view of the popularization of diverse exercise programs, both for medical testing and for physical conditioning, it is now also urgent to define the incidence of complications in order that appropriate prophylactic measures be instituted before preventable catastrophes throw the entire concept into unjustified disrepute.

MAJOR HAZARDS OF EXERCISE

In the patient with coronary heart disease (CHD), there are essentially two major complications which may be precipitated by exer-

* From the Cardiovascular Research Laboratories, Department of Nutrition, Harvard School of Public Health, and the Medical Clinics of the Peter Bent Brigham Hospital, Boston, Massachusetts. Supported in part by Grants HE-07776-06A1, 5T1-HE-5242, and PO1-HE-11306-03 from the National Institutes of Health, U. S. Public Health Service.

cise, namely, acute myocardial infarction and sudden death. There is no reason to surmise that exercise or sports activities affect the coronary vessel itself or favor intraluminal obstruction. It is, however, established that myocardial infarction may result from augmented cardiac work load when unsupported by increased coronary blood flow. In the patient with significant coronary vascular obstruction, the enhanced cardiac work load of exercise favors myocardial ischemia which may be sustained long enough to cause infarction.

Exercise may also provoke electrical instability of the myocardium, manifesting as ventricular arrhythmia leading to sudden death. The concept of electrical instability (3) has evolved from coronary care unit experience and postulates that acute myocardial ischemia promotes repetitive or early cycle ventricular premature beats (VPB's) and, at the same time, causes a reduction in threshold of the ventricular vulnerable period. Discharge of a VPB during the vulnerable period favors the development of ventricular fibrillation. In fact, the occurrence of any VPB's during an episode of myocardial ischemia is regarded as a possible harbinger of sudden death (4).

Already in 1927, Bourne (5) noted that exercise increased the frequency of VPB's in patients with CHD, but depressed ectopic activity in normals as well as in subjects with rheumatic heart disease. A similar conclusion was reached by Mann and Burchell (6). The frequent occurrence of VPB's with exercise in patients with CHD has been recently demonstrated (7). One hundred patients with CHD, sixty-nine with recent myocardial infarction and thirty-one with angina pectoris, performed graded treadmill exercise. Monitoring was carried out for a period of three minutes prior to the test. During the control period, 19 percent exhibited VPB's; exercise increased the incidence of ectopic beats to 43 percent. The increase of VPB's was from 8.3 to 16.2 percent for patients with angina pectoris and from 24.6 to 55.0 percent for those who had sustained recent myocardial infarction.

While exercise may precipitate both myocardial infarction and major arrythmias leading to sudden death, how frequently do these complications indeed occur? No certain data is available as to the incidence of catastrophic events in the exercising CHD patient. Some insight into this problem is provided by analysis of the type of patient subjected to exercise and the form of exercise employed.

EXERCISE OF THE PATIENT WITH
ACUTE MYOCARDIAL INFARCTION

This is not a hypothetical problem since as many as 25 percent of myocardial infarctions go unrecognized by both patient and physician (8). Such silent infarctions are not due to minor lesions. During a fourteen-year follow-up period in the prospective Framingham Study, silent infarcts posed the same threat of subsequent coronary attack and death as did symptomatic episodes of coronary occlusion (8). Presumably, patients with unrecognized infarcts have been fully active during the acute stage. Many of these so-called silent infarct patients may be the victims of sudden death. The magnitude of this occurrence is unascertainable.

The traditional, deeply held conviction of many physicians is that activity during acute myocardial infarction is frought with hazard. Current practice in treating acute myocardial infarction is guided by the concept that rest promotes healing of an injured organ. It is believed that activity may provoke fatal arrhythmias or predispose to congestive heart failure, cardiac rupture, or ventricular aneurysm formation. Support for this view stems from the remarkable findings of Jetter and White (9). Twenty percent of severly psychotic patients who succumbed to unrecognized myocardial infarction exhibited cardiac rupture. These patients remained fully active during the attack. In a nonpsychotic control group, the incidence was 3 percent. There is no other clinical evidence indicating deleterious effect of activity undertaken during the evolution of a myocardial infarction.

Experimental studies on this important subject are nearly equally sparse. In a small series of dogs subjected to coronary artery ligation, Sutton and Davis (10) noted that daily exercise led to ventricular aneurysm formation. However, this conclusion was based on five animals, four being exercised within three days of ligation. On the other hand, Thomas and Harrison (11) have suggested that early exercise is without hazard, and compared to complete rest, may be beneficial. They studied the effect of activity level upon mortality in rats that had been subjected to thermal injury of the myocardium. Control and exercised rats showed the same mortality, whereas complete restriction of activity in a small cage led to a significantly higher death rate. The most detailed study of this question was carried out by Lown and co-workers (12). Two groups of dogs with coronary artery ligation were compared as to the effects of exercise. One group was exercised beginning with the third day after ligation on a motorized treadmill twice daily for five weeks, while the control group was kept at complete rest during this period. The rigorous exercise program did not provoke major arrhythmia or sudden death. Even though the exercise was performed during the evolution of an acute myocardial infarction, the characteristic adaptation to physical training was observed, namely reduction in heart rate, cardiac index, and in blood levels of lactic acid. No cardiac rupture occurred; no aneurysms were noted. The size of infarction was identical in exercising and control animals.

It is difficult to extrapolate these results to man. The healthy animal with an artificially induced coronary occlusion at only one locus is hardly comparable to the patient whose disease has progressed over years and which results in a diffuse process usually involving the entire coronary tree. Furthermore, these studies were not carried out during the very acute initial days after coronary artery closure. At present, therefore, no evidence exists as to the danger of activity or exercise during acute myocardial infarction. If activity is indeed deleterious, the duration of the period of required rest is undetermined.

EXERCISE TESTING OF CHD PATIENTS

A large literature exists on the effect of limited exercise in individuals with known or suspected CHD. The reason for such exercise testing is to determine the presence or extent of CHD. It derives from a chance observation by Feil and Siegel (13) who noted that when a patient is having anginal pain, there are concomitant alterations in electrocardiogram. In 1936, Wood and co-workers (14) noted differences in the electrocardiographic responses to stair climbing of normal subjects as compared with patients having angina pectoris. Modern diagnostic exercise testing derives from the classic work of Master and Jaffe (15). The basic physiologic consideration underlying such tests is that the adequacy of coronary blood flow is related to the metabolic requirements of heart muscle cells. By increasing cardiac work, it is possible to expose inadequacies of coronary flow. The balance of supply and demand is being interpreted in terms of electrical activity of the heart, defined by deviation in ST segment.

The Master two-step test imposes a fixed and limited exercise load determined exclusively by the age and weight of the subject. There have been more than 50,000 such tests performed with a remarkable paucity of complications. Grossman and Grossman (16) have reported a single case of myocardial infarction. This occurred in a forty-two-year-old man who, four months earlier, had experienced severe and sustained substernal pain which was later considered to have been due to a "mild heart attack." Subsequent to this attack he experienced angina pectoris as well as angina decubitus. The resting electrocardiogram is described as "borderline." After eight trips over the two steps, he developed unusual and incapacitating dyspnea. At no time did he experience chest pressure or substernal pain. The electrocardiogram revealed paroxysms of ventricular tachycardia and a massive current of injury. This patient evolved, thereafter, changes of anterior wall myocardial infarction.

Arrhythmias have been noted with the Master test. Lloyd Thomas (17) reported a transient bout of ventricular fibrillation immediately after an exercise test in a patient with angina pectoris. Mattingly (18) noted two episodes of short lived junctional tachycardia as the sole complication of such testing. Miller and Pollard (19) encountered two short bursts of tachycardia, one junctional and the other perhaps ventricular. On the other hand, Robb and Marks (20) performed two-step exercise testing without any complications in 1659 applicants for insurance, half of whom had chest pain. Similarly, Brody (21) noted no complications except for an evanescent tachycardia in one lead in one of 756 patients subjected to a double Master two-step test. Lamb and Hiss (22), in 1851 individuals exercised on a two-step, observed no significant arrhythmia.

It can be concluded that exercise as prescribed by Master (23, 24), even in the patient with advanced CHD, is safe. The simple precautions recommended by Master are fully adequate to assure absence of complications.

SUBMAXIMAL AND MAXIMAL EXERCISE TESTING

The time integral of tension per beat remains relatively constant during exercise; the challenge to the coronary circulation, therefore, derives primarily from the increase in heart rate. The oxygen consumption of the heart per minute varies in proportion to the acceleration in rate (25). Unless the exercise is sufficiently severe, the heart rate is but minimally increased. In such circumstances, many patients with CHD will have normal responses. The Master two-step test produces an inadequate stress for many patients, since the level of exercise is arbitrarily fixed and is unrelated to the subject's level of physical conditioning. Exercise tests have, therefore, been introduced which achieve higher heart rates (25, 26). A motorized treadmill is employed, and the stress of exercise is graded.

Sheffield and Reeves (25) have determined the adequacy of exercise on the basis of heart rate, where the rate is forced to about 85 percent of the maximal predicted for the subject's age. They have noted no significant complications. Doyle and Kinch (27) have employed submaximal treadmill exercise testing. Over a thirteen-year period, they have performed 22,223 tests in 2437 males. Of this number, only 264 developed electrocardiographic and other manifestations consistent with CHD. They encountered no complications. Bruce and co-workers (28) have carried out 4000 treadmill tests and have encountered but a single major complication. These investigators have reported this complication in some detail. The patient was a forty-two-year-old man without known heart disease, with a normal electrocardiogram. Three years earlier a maximal graded exercise test resulted in a normal response. He reached ninety-seven seconds of stage four exercise (4.2 mph at grade of 16°), and stopped because of fatigue. There were no cardiac symptoms and no deviation in ST segment. Following a minor psychologic irritation, resulting from scalding with hot water while showering, he experienced marked fatigue and irritability. He was immediately seen by a physician. An electrocardiogram revealed an anterior wall current of injury. Within five minutes, ventricular tachycardia and ventricular fibrillation developed. He was promptly and effectively resuscitated. This patient thereupon evolved an anterior myocardial infarction and was left with a small apical ventricular aneurysm. A coronary angiogram taken six months later revealed a normal right coronary artery, a diseased anterior descending vessel, and occlusion of the left circumflex. It is noteworthy that this patient had a normal response to submaximal exercise.

Ellestad and associates (29) have carried out 4028 maximal capacity stress tests on a treadmill without encountering any deaths. In the 1000 patients they reported upon, of whom 266 had exercise induced ischemic electrocardiographic changes, 9 developed ventricular tachycardia, and in one patient the arrhythmia was sustained and required cardioversion. Two other patients had myocardial infarction temporally related to the test; both survived. Among five hundred patients with CHD exercised on a treadmill by Kattus and McAlpin (30), two developed ventricular fibrillation which was fatal in one. Hornstein and Bruce (31) defined the minimal incidence of major complication in such graded treadmill exercise as six per forty thousand tests. Of the six complications, four were due to myocardial infarction, and two were arrhythmia deaths.

Phibbs (32) has emphasized that there exists a time lag between imposition of exercise stress on the myocardium and the appearance of major arrhythmia or substantial ischemic changes in the electrocardiogram. In 787 tests he found 327 to be positive for ischemic heart disease. Of this latter number, 75, or 22.9 percent, demonstrated significant alterations only after completion of the treadmill exercise test. Three patients developed major complications, including massive current of injury and ventricular flutter, four to five minutes after termination of exercise. The steady increase in heart rate of multistage exercise precludes emergence of ventricular arrhythmia during the exercise because of rate overdrive. The electrocardiogram, therefore, is an inadequate guide to the level of exercise. Upon resumption of rest, and especially recumbency, arrhythmias may emerge. Phibbs (31) therefore suggests an interrupted series of exercises, namely each progressive increase in work load is to be followed by a rest period.

EXERCISE CONDITIONING

Active physical conditioning of the patient with CHD is gaining wide medical sanction (33). Complications during programs of supervised jogging, swimming, calisthenics, and other sports are thus beginning to appear in the medical literature. Cantwell and Fletcher (34) encountered complications in two patients participating in an organized exercise program. One patient, a forty-year-old man, developed severe substernal pain and an acute diaphragmatic infarction while attempting to jog one and one-half miles three weeks after entering an exercise conditioning program. The second patient, a fifty-one-year-old, played volleyball and ran 440 yards when he collapsed. A physician running behind found him cyanotic, pulseless, with dilated pupils. He was successfully resuscitated. It is of interest that the electrocardiogram and serum enzymes failed to show the characteristic pattern of acute myocardial infarction. Pyfer and Doane (35) report on a sixty-one-year-old man with a history of two prior myocardial infarctions who had been actively participating in a group rehabilitation program for six months. He was able to run a mile three days weekly. On three separate occasions he was tested on a bicycle ergometer with maximal exercise and showed no abnormal physical or electrocardiographic findings. During forward bending exercises, he experienced cardiac arrest. Resuscitation by defibrillation, which was carried out in the gymnasium, was successful. This patient also exhibited no sequential serum enzyme or electrocardiographic alterations consistent with myocardial infarction.

Frick and Katila (36) subjected seven male patients, within two to four months after myocardial infarction, to three periods weekly of ergometer exercise training. There was some improvement in hemodynamics and no complications. Similarly, Clausen and co-workers (37) trained nine male patients on an electrically braked bicycle ergometer, eight of whom had sustained myocardial infarction in the past. No complications were observed.

While mild noncompetitive exercises, such as running, swimming, and calisthenics, have been the rule in the thousands of reconditioning centers now operating in Europe and the United States, strenuous exertion and competitive sports have been precluded for the patient with overt CHD. However, Gottheimer (38), in Israel, has employed the most arduous isometric and endurance exercises since 1955 for rehabilitating cardiacs. Until 1964, 3000 such patients had participated in programs of reconditioning. Of this number, 1461 had CHD, and about half had sustained acute myocardial infarction. It is of interest that subjects with previous myocardial infarction were able to run 11 km in from fifty-eight to eighty minutes. Only one beginner died in a sports event. Patients were subjected to a gradual conditioning process over several months of daily workouts. Of the patients with ischemic heart disease, 1103 remained under observation for five years. In this group there were forty-nine deaths, of which forty, or 3.6 percent, were due to cardiac causes. Gottheimer suggests that the anticipated mortality in a similar non-exercising group would be around 12 percent. A similar conclusion was reached by Hellerstein (39) based on rehabilitation through exercise conditioning of 245 patients with angina pectoris or myocardial infarction.

The reported experience suggests that when cardiac patients are closely supervised and there are long preparatory periods of mild warm-up with strength and endurance promoting exercises, there is no significant hazard in strenuous sports. Furthermore, it appears that major complications, such as the occurrence of fatal arrhythmia, are not predictable by currently employed methods.

UNSUPERVISED EXERCISES

What is the hazard for the middle-aged, unconditioned male who decides to partake of some strenuous, unrehearsed exertion? There is no information on the potential danger of such an impulsive activity. Anyone residing in the northern lattitudes, however, is familiar with the brimming obituary columns following a snowstorm. That ambitious exercise programs in the unconditioned, middle-aged or elderly male are probably dangerous is also indicated by diverse reports. For example, in less than twelve months in Orange County, California, there have been at least eight deaths of men in jogging clothes or of men starting new physical activity (40).

There are also occasional communications in the medical literature of sudden deaths during sports activities among young individuals. Generally, a medical history provides no relevant clues, and routine postmortem examination affords no special insights. Recently, James *et al.* (41)reported on two such fatalities. The first was an eighteen-year-old boy who died suddenly while playing football. He was known to have had bradycardia in the past. A careful pathologic study revealed medial hyperplasia of the sinus node artery with complete occlusion at several points in this vessel's course. There were foci of old and recent hemorrhage, and degeneration in the sinus node. The second victim was a fifteen-year-old boy who complained of feeling sick while wrestling, turned blue, and expired. The pathologic findings were similar to that noted in the first patient. The basis for these morphologic alterations is unclear. Death was assumed to be due to arrhythmia.

It should be noted, for the sake of completeness, that there is a rare patient who, on minimal exertion, develops ventricular tachycardia which may last for minutes or even days. Both complete remission and sudden death have been recorded (42, 43). Recently, beta blocking drugs have been shown to prevent exercise-induced recurrence of arrhythmia (44).

OVERALL ASSESSMENT

A review of the literature and of our own experience indicates that exercise may precipitate major arrhythmia; at times it may even result in death. However, the hazard is much over rated. Whether serious complications occur depends upon three factors: the nature and extent of coronary pathology, the type of exercise undertaken, and the state of conditioning of the patient. There exists no evidence whether activity or exercise is hazardous for patients who are in the recovery phase of acute myocardial infarction. If exercise is indeed injurious, there is no certainty as to the duration of the period of rest during convalescence. Exercise testing for ischemic heart disease over a two-step, as prescribed by Master, is safe and is remarkably free of any significant complications. Multistage exercise on treadmill carries a small hazard which is generally unpredictable. Exercise conditioning is remarkably safe, even for the patient with far advanced CHD, if the program is graduated and there is close medical supervision. Exercise may result in complication when it is undertaken casually and sporadically by the unconditioned, middle-aged individual, especially when the exercise is strenuous and competitive. Buoyed by a sense of well-being, which exercise may provide, and propelled by exuberant pride, which competition sets in motion, exertion may be carried beyond the capacity of a restricted coronary circulation. No precautions will prove adequate against such episodic human overindulgence. The only possible answer resides in increased popular education and provision of well staffed and supervised facilities for initiation of exercise conditioning.

REFERENCES

1. Paul, O.: In Fox, S. M., III: Physical activity and coronary heart disease. *Amer J Cardiol, 23*:298-306, 1969.
2. Fox, S. M., and Haskell, W. L.: Physical activity and the prevention of coronary heart disease. *Bull NY Acad Med, 44*:950-967, 1968.
3. Lown, B., Klein, M., and Hershberg, P.: Coronary and precoronary care. *Amer J Med, 46*:705-724, 1969.
4. Lown, B., Kosowsky, B. D., and Klein, M. D.: Pathogenesis, prevention and treatment of arrhythmias in myocardial infarction. Circulation, *39:(suppl. IV)*:261-270, 1969.
5. Bourne, G.: An attempt at the clinical classification of premature ventricular beats. *Quart J Med, 20*:219-243, 1927.
6. Mann, R. H., and Burchell, H. B.: Premature ventricular contractions and exercise. *Proc Staff Mayo Clinic, 27*:383-389, 1952.
7. Lown, B., Kosowsky, B. D., and Whiting, R.: Exposure of electrical instability in coronary artery disease by exercise stress. *Circulation, 39 (suppl. III)*:118, 1969.
8. Kannel, W. B., McNamara, P. M., Feinleib, M. *et al.*: Unrecognized myocardial infarction. *Geriatrics, 25*:75-87, 1970.
9. Jetter, W. W., and White, P. D.: Rupture of the heart in patients in mental institutions. *Ann Intern Med, 21*:783-802, 1944.
10. Sutton, D. C., and Davis, M. D.: Effect of exercise on experimental cardiac infarction. *Arch Intern Med, 48*:1118-1125, 1931.
11. Thomas, W. C., and Harrison, T. R.: Effect of artificial restriction of activity on the recovery of rats with experimental myocardial injury. *Amer J Med Sci, 208*:436-450, 1944.
12. Kaplinsky, E., Hood, W. B., Jr., McCarthy, B. *et al.*: Effects of physical training in dogs with coronary artery ligation. *Circulation, 37*:556-565, 1968.
13. Feil, H., and Siegel, M. L.: Electrocardiographic changes during attacks of angina pectoris. *Amer J Med Sci, 175*:255-260, 1928.
14. Wood, F. C., and Wolferth, C. C.: Angina pectoris; clinical and electrocardiographic phenomena of attack and their comparison with effects of experimental temporary coronary occlusion. *Arch Intern Med, 47*:339-365, 1931.
15. Master, A. M., and Jaffe, H. L.: Electrocardiographic changes after exercise in angina pectoris. *J Mount Sinai Hosp NY, 7*:629-632, 1941.

16. Grossman, L. A., and Grossman, M.: Myocardial infarction precipitated by Master two step test. *JAMA, 158*:179-180, 1955.

17. Lloyd, T. H. G.: The exercise electrocardiogram in patients with cardiac pain. *Brit Heart J, 23*:561-577, 1961.

18. Mattingly, T. W., Fancher, P. S., Bauer, F. L. *et al.*: The value of the double standard 2-step exercise tolerance test in detecting coronary disease in a follow-up study of 1,000 military personnel. Research Report, Army Medical Service Graduate School 21-54, Walter Reed Medical Center, Washington, D. C., September, 1954.

19. Miller, P. B., and Pollard, L. W.: Paroxysmal tachycardia after exercise. *Circulation, 26*:363-372, 1962.

20. Robb, G. P., and Marks, H. H.: Latent coronary artery disease: Determination of its presence and severity by the exercise electrocardiogram. *Amer J Cardiol, 13*:603-618, 1964.

21. Brody, A. J.: Master two-step test in clinically unselected patients. *JAMA, 171*:1195-1198, 1959.

22. Lamb, L. E., and Hiss, R. G.: Influence of exercise on premature contractions. *Amer J Cardiol, 10*:209-216, 1962.

23. Master, A. M., and Rosenfeld, I.: Monitored and post exercise two-step test: Detection of silent coronary heart disease and differential diagnosis of chest pain. *JAMA, 190*:494-500, 1964.

24. Master, A. M., and Rosenfeld, I.: Two-step exercise test: Current status after twenty-five years. *Mod Conc Cardiov Dis, 36*:19-24, 1967.

25. Sheffield, L. T., and Reeves, T. J.: Graded exercise in the diagnosis of angina pectoris. *Med Conc Cardiov Dis, 34*:1-6, 1965.

26. Doan, A. E., Peterson, D., Blackman, J. R. *et al.*: Myocardial ischemia after maximal exercise in healthy men. *Amer Heart J, 69*:11-21, 1965.

27. Doyle, J. T., and Kinch, S. H.: The prognosis of an abnormal electrocardiographic stress test. *Circulation, 41*:545-554, 1970.

28. Bruce, A. R., Hornstein, T. R., and Blackman, J. R.: Myocardial infarctions after normal responses to maximal exercise. *Circulation, 38*:552-558, 1968.

29. Ellestad, M., Allen, W., Wan, C. K. M. *et al.*: Maximal treadmill stress testing for cardiovascular evaluation. *Circulation, 39*:517-522, 1969.

30. Kattus, A. A., and McAlpin, R. N.: Diagnosis, medical and surgical management of coronary insufficiency. *Ann Intern Med, 69*:115-136, 1968.

31. Hornstein, T. R., and Bruce, R. A.: Stress testing, safety precautions and cardiovascular health. *J Occup Med, 10*:640-648, 1968.

32. Phibbs, B., Holmes, R. W., and Lowe, C. R.: Transient myocardial ischemia: The Significance of dyspnea. *Amer J Med Sci, 256*:210-221, 1968.

33. Hellerstein, H. K., Hornstein, T. R., Goldbarg, A. N. *et al.*: In Brest, A. N., and Moyer, J. H. (Eds.): *The influence of active conditioning*

upon coronary atherosclerosis, *Atherosclerotic Vascular Disease, Hahne-mann Symposium.* New York, Appleton County Crofts, 1967, pp. 115-129.

34. Cantwell, J. D., and Fletcher, G. F.: Cardiac complications while jogging. *JAMA, 210*:130-131, 1969.

35. Pyfer, H. R., and Doane, B. L.: Cardiac arrest during exercise training: Report of a successfully treated case attributed to preparedness. *JAMA, 210*:101-102, 1969.

36. Frick, M. H., and Katila, M.: Hemodynamic consequences of physical training after myocardial infarction. *Circulation, 37*:192-202, 1968.

37. Clausen, J. P., Larsen, O. A., and Trap-Jensen, J.: Physical training in the management of coronary artery disease. *Circulation, 40*:143-154, 1969.

38. Gottheimer, V.: Long range strenuous sports training for cardiac reconditioning and rehabilitation. *Amer J Cardiol, 22*:426-435, 1968.

39. Hellerstein, H. K.: Exercise therapy in coronary disease. *Bull NY Acad Med, 44*:1028-1047, 1968.

40. Fox, S.: Personal communication based on a report from Ronald H. Silvester, M. D., Ranchos Amigos Hospital, Downey, California.

41. James, T., Froggatt, P., and Marshall, T. K.: Sudden death in young athletes. *Ann Intern Med, 67*:1013-1021, 1967.

42. Wilson, F. N., Wishart, S. W., Macleod, A. O. *et al.*: Clinical type of paroxysmal tachycardia of ventricular origin in which paroxysms are induced by exertion. *Amer Heart J, 8*:155-169, 1932.

43. Dimond, E. G., and Hayes, W. L.: Benign paroxysmal ventricular tachycardia: Report of a case. *Ann Intern Med, 53*:1255-1260, 1960.

44. Taylor, R. R., and Halliday, E. J.: Beta adrenergic blockade in the treatment of exercise-induced paroxysmal ventricular tachycardia. *Circulation, 32*:778-781, 1965.

Chapter 11

SUMMARY PANEL ON GUIDELINES

LAWRENCE A. GOLDING, WILLIAM C. DAY, LORING B. ROWELL,
HOWARD G. KNUTTGEN, WILLIAM B. KANNEL, EUGENE Z. HIRSCH,
AND PER-OLOF ÅSTRAND

Dr. Morse: In order to return the theme of the Symposium to the subject of exercise programs for essentially well people, the Symposium will be concluded by the return of our main speakers, with a short presentation crystalizing their thoughts and including some of the answers to questions which have been raised. A reasonable point of view would be that of a small group some place, some place not connected with an academic community, some place that perhaps has some modest facility for exercising groups—some place that has people who are interested in developing exercising programs. At least we could start with enthusiasm and leadership. If we start from this hypothetical situation, can we then ask our speakers how, in their opinion, is the best way to construct an exercise program.

EXERCISE CLASSES
(Lawrence A. Golding)

Dr. Golding, if I were now to start with the idea of an exercise program, what would you give me for advice as to what specific sets of exercises and what doses of these exercises do you think we ought to offer?

Dr. Golding: That is not an easy question and cannot be answered by a simple statement. I know those of you who are YMCA physical directors could do as good a job of answering this as I can because your major role is to get people to exercise. One can suggest exercises, but unless people *do* them, they are of no value. You've got to have exercises that not only people will start doing, but will continue doing. First of all, the success of any program depends upon the leadership. Any physical director can tell you that if you have a successful program, you must have a successful leader. Individuals

[213]

do not basically like to exercise, and there are very few people who can exercise by themselves. There are very few who have the discipline that will enable them to go out every day and exercise alone. Most individuals need to have some kind of pressure, some kind of discipline, to keep them interested and exercising. This means that someone has to encourage them; someone has to lead them; someone has to tell them what to do; someone has to show them how much they are improving and how much good it is doing.

Dr. Morse: Taking leadership as our basic requirement, now what do you do?

Dr. Golding: I think it was pointed out that most people who become interested in fitness are not particularly well-skilled athletically, so the general fitness program that you see in the YMCA is probably best for most people. Being good physical educators, we should stress a well balanced program so that we are getting some skeletal muscle development as well as cardiovascular fitness. Of course the major emphasis, as this conference has shown, is on aerobic power or the development of the heart, circulation, and lungs so that they become more efficient. This involves mainly running and swimming. Running is the easiest cardiovascular activity because it needs no equipment and it does not need a great deal of skill. Everybody can run, although not everybody can swim.

Dr. Morse: How many times a week do you exercise?

Dr. Golding: Obviously, if you could exercise seven days a week, you would get better results than if you exercised five days a week. Five days a week would give you better results than three days a week, but it is pretty difficult to get people to exercise every day. Likewise it is difficult to get people to exercise even five days a week. So, I think that somewhere we have to be realistic and say that you can do a good exercise program and get good results with only three days a week.

Dr. Morse: What should be included in the program of exercise?

Dr. Golding: I think that some kind of a warm-up period, which includes the type of exercises that you often see in the Y involving a lot of rhythmical, swinging type of movement, is desirable. Then there needs to be some skeletal muscle development, which includes the typical calisthenics. Four or five well chosen calisthenics could exercise each major muscle group of the body. Then I would concentrate on running for cardiovascular fitness. I do not believe that you have to run ten miles to attain it. You can become very fit running no more than two miles if you work on intensity instead of distance. Some studies have indicated that interval training produces better oxygen uptake values than long continuous running.

A reasonable kind of program, therefore, would involve a class with a good leader, giving warm-up, rhythmical type of activity, followed by some kind of calisthenic activity, and concluded with a running schedule, including interval work done three times a week with a minimum of thirty minutes each time.

MEDICAL ADVISORS
(William C. Day)

Dr. Morse: One problem is the distressing lack of expert opinion and expert advice necessary for these programs. If we are working in a small town, where can we find somebody who can watch our program along with us, and keep us from falling into poor and possibly dangerous habits?

Mr. Day: Possibly the best people to ask would be the physicians who are already involved in an advisory capacity in the program. I took a survey which included asking these physicians what "turned them off" and what "turned them on" when a physical educator approached them. We came up with a few "principles."

The first thing is that the physical director should not wait for the medical doctor to come to him. I know of at least one physical director who said that he could not start a program because the medical people in his community would not support it, and none of them had offered to help. So, the first thing one might do is to call one of them and at least make the attempt to confront him. I think there will be doctors in your community who are not interested in exercise. You should not be discouraged if the first doctor with whom you talk refuses to help or, because of time and other things, can't help. Don't give up at that point because you will, sooner or later, find one or more who are willing to help.

I asked one of our doctors in Cambridge what would "turn him off" if I, as a physical educator, came to him and asked for his support. His reply was "selling the program in a rather sensational way, as some faddist health magazines do." So don't go into his office armed with the latest editions of some of these magazines, and say that you have found a way to cure cancer and you need his help.

Finally, I really think that your attitude as a physical educator toward the fitness program is the key. If you look upon the physical fitness program as being just another program in the YMCA or you are seeking the medical doctor's aid because it is the thing to do, then I don't know of any doctor who would be willing to support you. But, if you go to him, having done a little bit of homework, you will know what exercise can and cannot do. You can tell him that you need him in order for this program to succeed. Without medical support you are not interested in administering a program because you know that without medical backing and medical advice the program will ultimately fail. If you sincerely solicit his support, I don't know of too many doctors who would turn you down.

PHYSIOLOGY

(Loring B. Rowell)

Dr. Morse: A reasonable question which one of the participants may voice is "What is it that is happening inside me, especially to my heart?" Dr. Rowell, can you answer this question?

Dr. Rowell: A rearrangement of the Fick equation is

$$\dot{V}_{O_2} = \text{H.R.} \times \text{S.V.} \times \text{AVO}_2$$

where $\dot{V}_{O_2}$ = oxygen consumption

H.R. = heart rate

S.V. = stroke volume

A V O_2 $\triangle$ = arterio - venous oxygen difference

Therefore the oxygen consumption equals the rate of the pump (HR) times the volume pumped with each beat (SV) times the amount of oxygen that is extracted (A V O_2 $\triangle$). I pointed out that the maximum range of response to these three variables determines the maximum range of response of oxygen consumption. When someone is physically conditioned, his maximum oxygen consumption is increased by an amount which depends on his age, etc. and his initial state of physical condition. What is always increased in terms of the cardiovascular parameters of oxygen transport listed above is the stroke volume. The heart pumps more blood per beat, i.e. its efficiency improves. The capacity to increase oxygen extraction (A V O$_2$ $\triangle$) may also increase. If the individual is relatively fit to begin with, the major change is in stroke volume so that the product of heart rate and stroke volume gives a slightly greater maximum cardiac output. In unfit subjects the increase in AVO$_2$$\triangle$ contributes relatively more to the increased capacity and may equal the contribution of increased stroke volume. Presumably part of the increased A V O$_2$ $\triangle$ is due to distribution of a greater fraction of total blood flow to working muscle where most O$_2$ is being extracted from blood. Thus, more blood reaches muscle because more is pumped, but also more of what is pumped may reach muscle as well.

TESTING
(Howard G. Knuttgen)

Dr. Morse: Dr. Knuttgen, how could we initially test and subsequently evaluate what these people are doing throughout the program?

Dr. Knuttgen: Dr. Rowell has just pointed out that the heart rate response to exercise gives a good indication of the capacity of the circulatory system and, therefore, the body's capacity to deal with exercise stress. He also pointed out that it is an easy physiological parameter to measure. If I were organizing an exercise program, I would use either a step test or a bicycle ergometer to test the participants at the beginning of the program and then retest them throughout the program. The step test and the bicycle ergometer test establish a known and controllable work intensity. If I used a step test I would measure heart rate during recovery. I would prefer, however, to test the participants with the aid of a bicycle ergometer, one which provided an accurate measure of work. For equipment I would need only a bicycle ergometer (some of which can be obtained for a few hundred dollars), a stop-watch, and a metronome. I would determine steady state heart rate reaction to work at predetermined intensities. I would remember that body size is an important factor in determining work capacity, and I would interpret the results in terms of some measurement of size, such as body weight.

If I wanted to give additional interest to the measurement for the sake of the participant, I would predict maximum oxygen uptake with the use of the nomogram of Åstrand (*Acta Physiol Scand*, Vol. 49, Suppl. 169, 1960).

I would recognize that my exercise program was unique and that the levels of stress for the participants involved were dependent on a number of factors, such as the activities I had chosen, the pace I set, and the enthusiasm of the participants. I would, therefore, not expect to find standards in the literature which I could apply to my program, but I would begin to gather data from the results of the tests I gave and develop my own standards for (a) the initial level of exercise I would recommend for new participants, and (b) to determine if I really were aiding the participant to improve the functional capacity of his circulatory system.

MEDICAL SCREENING
(William B. Kannel)

Dr. Morse: It might be unwise to exercise every subject who applies for a general exercise program. Dr. Kannel, could you give us a short list of things to measure in these subjects, and could you tell us what the limits are for each test, that would make you suggest the patient *not* be put into a general exercise program?

Dr. Kannel: At the outset we all have to confess that we are dealing in the realm of the probable rather than the certain, and we really have no data on which to make dogmatic assertions. I think most of us are concerned with general exercise programs recommended for middle-aged and flabby men who are in general highly vulnerable to coronary attacks. Our job, it seems to me, is to pick out the ones who are most vulnerable and likely to get into trouble. Here it is simply a matter of estimating the probability of their being vulnerable to a high degree and therefore the probability of their getting into trouble. Most of us are fearful of the possibility of lethal consequences and hence, the focus on the cardiovascular implications of unrestricted, unaccustomed exercise. It seems to me that this necessitates an evaluation of coronary vulnerability in particular, to detect those who are likely to have advanced through silent coronary artery disease. The mere fact that the patient can go through a general physical examination and show no symptoms of heart disease does *not* guarantee that he will escape difficulty.

Consequently we should determine if the individual has hypertension (arbitrarily a level of 160/95 or greater), if he has an elevated cholesterol level (260 mg% or greater), or some impairment of glucose tolerance (a 2-hr level of 160 mg or greater). If he has any one of these atherogenic traits, it would seem reasonable to require that such a person have a resting ECG. If that is normal, then an exercise ECG should be obtained before he is certified for a general exercise program. If he has abnormalities of the exercise ECG, he still, it seems to me, would be eligible for a *properly supervised restricted* exercise program which may do him a lot of good, but unrestricted exercise could be dangerous. In fact, if the candidate has any two of the aforementioned hallmarks of increased vulnerability to coronary heart disease, he probably should be put on a restricted exercise program, even if his ECG at rest or post-exercise is normal.

Dr. Morse: What kind of ECG abnormalities will we look for?

Dr. Kannel: I think intraventricular block, left ventricular hypertrophy, certainly an unrecognized myocardial infarction, and post-exercise ECG ST depression ought to exclude the individual from a general exercise program. Some authorities would also consider multiple premature ventricular beats and paroxysmal tachycardia as possible exclusions. Certainly persons with atrial fibrillation probably should be excluded.

Evaluation of fitness and related factors is certainly indicated. Poor fitness is an indication for exercise, but I believe it is also an indication to proceed with caution. Such persons are vulnerable to sudden death. Those sedentary persons who are obese, have a rapid resting pulse rate, perform badly on dynomometry, or are quite breathless after exercise testing should have a post-exercise ECG before allowed unrestricted exercise. They should certainly also have the blood pressure and cholesterol and glucose tolerance measured. It is important to emphasize that persons who go into these programs are quite sedentary and often obese. They should be encouraged to lose weight. If they smoke heavily, they should be encouraged to stop.

RESTRICTED EXERCISE PROGRAM

(Eugene Z. Hirsch)

Dr. Morse: Dr. Kannel now has separated out a group of people who are not in general exercise programs. This group is very special, and we have not had too much experience with it. Dr. Hirsch, what are the few basic "do's" and "don'ts" about a group with known heart disease which we might consider exercising?

Dr. Hirsch: Physical activity must be treated as a normal, desirable component of daily human activity. Restoring or inducing the fit state can be accomplished safely. Fitness is relative and must be individualized. One must promote enthusiasm, but discourage competition and faddism. Particularly prone to these things are the cardiac patients who have a deeply vested interest in their therapy. One should aim to educate the patient to be an accurate intuitive judge of his own energy expenditure and physical and cardiac ability. After undergoing a reasonable period of instruction and coaching, I think it becomes obvious that the patient can be very sensitive to these things and can help himself by extending his activity judiciously.

The type of dynamic, large muscle group exercise is not critical, but standard exercise procedures must be included, as a continuing point of reference. Time taken to train is *not* critical. A patient can even start training *below* his work capacity. It may take time for the patient to go even beyond what he is capable of doing when he comes into the program. The patient may take from three to six months to accomplish the fitness level that he might be capable of reaching in two months. It is also advisable to carry out the first two weeks of training without significant stress, to allow the patient to acclimatize to the entire procedure.

I feel that a training program should screen patients into groups in which the limiting factors are (a) untrained muscles, or (b) myocardial ischemia. The second group should be tested initially with and without medications. Various medications have been mentioned by some of the speakers; nitroglycerin, beta blockers, and combinations. Patients with angina should be placed on the appropriate therapy in conjunction with supervised training and followed closely during the initial month or two of their training. In coronary patients we use nitroglycerine in small doses, as frequently as necessary, to the point of tolerance. Even in the absence of pain, we use 3 mg every eight to ten minutes during training sessions.

Training sessions consist of periods of warm-up, peak activity, tapering off, and relaxation. Warm-up in angina patients is particularly important in that many patients have "walk through" angina. If they warm up slowly, they may have angina initially, but after it leaves, the patients may then go on to exercise more vigorously without the recurrence of angina. Tapering off is particularly important to avoid dangerous bradycardias which may occur after the sudden cessation of exercise. Angina patients should engage first in short duration exercise (less than 2 min) with intervening rest periods so that you can monitor them.

Frequent personal contact must be built into the program. All the advice that you offer the patient must be given with recognition of the fact that reconditioning (including diet, no smoking, adequate sleep, etc.) is a long-term situation requiring adjustment and cannot be done all at once. Physical training is dangerous, I believe, for the patient with conorary disease if the functioning aspects of the patient have not been assessed and if physician supervision of particularly angina patients is not included at the outset. Eventually, these people may continue on their own, but initially a physician should supervise.

GENERAL CONSIDERATIONS
(Per-Olof Åstrand)

Dr. Morse: We would very much like to have Dr. Åstrand summarize where he feels we all stand in the field of exercise. Dr. Chapman, in his first remarks explained that Dr. Åstrand has had the first word in much of what we have discussed in the last couple of days. We would be honored if Dr. Åstrand would give us the last word in exercise and the heart today.

Dr. Åstrand: Mr. Chairman, ladies and gentlemen: I am in a very good position at the end of the Symposium. I do not have to answer any questions, and furthermore, I leave for Sweden soon, so I will be safe. I am happy that I had started to exercise before the meeting because otherwise I could have been scared to death by some of the things that could happen to me. I will end with more philosophical aspects.

I will not try to review the modern way of life. You know very well what it is all about. Maybe you have seen the article by Forbes in the *New England Journal of Medicine,* 1968, where he emphasized that the remaining lifetime in 1900 was 46.3 years; in 1954, 66.7; in 1964, 66.9. It has leveled off evidently with a tendency to decline again. One who celebrated his fiftieth anniversary in the year 1900 became almost as old as the one who is fifty years of age today. Certainly there are many diseases, for instance, infectious diseases, and other hazards of life which have been reduced or eliminated, but on the other hand, you have other factors which are a threat to life, particularly cardiovascular disease. So, one cannot avoid the thought that our modern way of life could be one important factor for this situation and in a way, the main determinants of longevity are now more cultural than medical.

It has taken one million years or more to develop the Homo sapiens, and I don't think anything has happened for the last half century as far as genetic adaptation is concerned. So, if a pediatric doctor could examine a child born in the Stone Age, or a child born today, there wouldn't be any difference; both were constructed for activity.

For optimal function you need activity. You can adapt to various situations. You are all familiar with what happens in prolonged exposure to heat, to cold, to high altitudes, to exercise. The drawback is the ease with which you adapt to this situation. From physiological measurement, you can notice marked changes taking place even if you subjectively may not realize so. I will not now discuss patients. I think still there are some 150 to maybe 170 million Americans who are not patients, and we should consider them too.

I would like to start with back troubles because that is one thing that has nothing to do with this Symposium, but diseases in the spinal column rank very high on the list of common diseases. They are responsible for many days of sick leave and for much suffering. Therefore, I think it is important to include some activity which trains your trunk muscles. It will not heal your back, or it may not influence the inevitable changes in the spinal column that come with age, but they may prevent the symptoms caused by the occurrence of a weak back.

I pointed out that the joints should have some activity since there is much evidence that the movements increase the thickness of the cartilage and improve the exchange of nutriments. In my opinion you should avoid violent twisting and bending. I am not too interested in flexibility myself. I am not interested to try and reach the floor with stretched legs because I am clever enough to bend my knees if I want to reach for something.

I want to emphasize nutritional aspects just briefly. As time goes by, the weight of the Swedes and Americans increases more rapidly than the number of inhabitants, if you understand what I mean. I just want to emphasize that if you walk or run 2 km a day, that is one and one-quarter miles, it consumes about 100 kcal a day. That means that, after ten years, 365,000 kcal would be consumed, and that corresponds to about 130 pounds of adipose tissue.

So over long periods of time I think that exercise is essential, and also, as pointed out by Mayer and co-workers, the appetite functions more effectively in the physically active than in the inactive one. I love food, and I want to eat very much, but then I have to use up the calories. I don't like to go hungry often; this you eventually have to do if you are habitually inactive.

In Sweden, at least, it is emphasized that our food habits are geared to an intake of about 2,500 kcal per day, and with that high caloric intake, you are safe as far as proteins, vitamins, and iron supply is concerned. But now we have many "low caloric consumers," particularly women and elderly men. They run the risk that their supply of various nutrients becomes too small. Therefore, it is emphasized that the low caloric consumers should be stimulated to become "high caloric consumers" by regular exercise, and therefore they all may eat more, and automatically it will cover the supply of essential nutrients.

So you have the paradoxical situation that maybe two thirds of the population of the world are suffering from malnutrition because food is not available. Then you have one third of the population also suffering from malnutrition because they are physically inactive. This is, in many points, just quoting Mayer and co-workers. I think it is wonderful that here you have one aspect in favor of regular physical activity which has nothing to do directly with cardiovascular disease. On the other hand, many of the common diseases, such as diabetes, constipation, and iron-deficiency anemia, are more common among the low-caloric consumers.

In Sweden we have not this legal aspect: I don't think it could ever happen that a doctor, a coach, or any teacher of physical education could be sued because a person following his advice had a myocardial infarction. It just does not happen.

It has been claimed, and I know many doctors who emphasize, that before going to an exercise program, you should go and see your physician. I take the other look. I am convinced that regular physical activity is beneficial from many points of view. After all, I have only one heart, and I want to take good care of it! So, to be a little bit provocative, anyone who is doubtful about his state of health, should of course consult his physician. But, in principle, there is less risk in activity than in continuous inactivity. So, in a nutshell, my opinion is that it is more advisable to pass a careful medical examination if one intends to maintain a sedentary life, in order to establish whether one's state of health is good enough to stand the inactivity.

Therefore, I could as well say that if I were struck by heart disease as a citizen of the United states of America, I should go to my doctor and say to him, "Why didn't you tell me that I should start exercising?" This question has another practical aspect. In Sweden we now have many television programs where we emphasize the importance of regular physical exercise. Now if you had the same here and were successful, one hundred million Americans might want to start exercising. As far as I can see you would not have physicians enough to examine all of the individuals who would want to start a training program. Furthermore, it is also critical that there does not exist, in my opinion, a health examination which is foolproof. So even very advanced examinations, including work tests, give quite a number of false positive as well as false negative diagnoses.

I emphasize again, I am not discussing cardiovascular patients. In a conference in Sweden it was said, "Okay, take the electrocardiogram, but don't care about it now, just put it in the file somewhere. It will be nice for the future to have it." It is an actual fact that if you have the sixty-year-old man without symptoms, without any complaints, about 45 percent of them will have ECG changes which are the same as those found in ischemic heart disease according to the Minnesota code. Among the women, amazingly enough, 50 percent of the sixty-year-old women would have the same changes. Should the doctor tell one half of the middle-aged population not to take part in exercise and the other half that they should exercise? Of course I am provocative, but I think I have earned the right to be so.

My program of exercise must be the perfect program! I take my car to a golf course, but I do not play golf. Because it is wonderful terrain, I warm up, jog, and walk for five minutes uphill (only 25 steps but at maximum speed) because I think it is good training for trunk muscles and leg muscles. I walk down and repeat about five, six, seven times. People think I have a poor memory but I don't care. Here I rely on adenosine triphosphate and creatine phosphate, so I am not bothering my heart too much. It could be omitted from the program, I think. Then there is the conditioning of the cardiovascular system with three minutes of running; probably I could run this distance within two or two and one-half minutes, but I think it is as effective to do it in three minutes. Resting, jogging, and walking, and again running are then repeated, and after about one-half hour I am back to my car and go home. I try to devote three thirty-minute sessions per week to such training. In almost every Swedish community they are preparing such simple tracks. Eventually there will be tracks in the forest and electric lighting. It is dark in Sweden in winter. So, for twenty-four hours a day you can utilize it for walking, jogging, or running, or cross-country skiing in winter.

It was emphasized that you should have a choice of alternatives, for instance, swimming, bicycling, etc. It should not be too severe a load. We claim that one should exercise to a high enough level that conversation should not be easy and smooth, but if you are running or otherwise exercising, a conversation should not be impossible because of the respiratory response to lactic acid. It is a guide that you should still be able to speak a few words at a time even in your running or swimming or bicycling.

If I was a teacher at the YMCA or in a school, I should have a bicycle ergometer. In Sweden now it is compulsory in every school to have the bicycle. That is a joint effort between teachers in biology and in physical education. Maybe we should say that our generation is a lost generation as far as physical activity is concerned, excluding we who are gathered here in the hall, of course. So we have, maybe, to concentrate on the next generation and teach them the principles and try to teach them that physical activity is part of culture. I would also like to emphasize active recreation. It is important in my opinion. It has nothing to do with training, but it is a hobby where muscles are moving. There are more and more evidences that when working, as you know, the muscle spindles are stimulated and send impulses particularly to the reticular formation. I believe that those impulses from the muscles reach important parts of the brain. Dr. Chapman mentioned exercise as a tranquilizer, and this impulse traffic might be part of the explanation.

As for golf, I am quite positive. Firstly it makes the low calorie consumer a high calorie consumer in a way. It is not so critical if you walk slow or fast or even run. The distance is the most important factor. If you then want to train, why not leave the golf stick at home sometimes.

So, in summary, I am very positive for regular exercise and do enjoy exercise, but in a way, I don't care whether I live longer or shorter. So it is a question of, as has been said before, to add life to years rather than to add years to life. One guide is that you should have a physical conditioning program demanding more effort than the routine job. For anyone with a habitual sedentary job, it might be enough to walk, but those who are lumberjacks should actually train rather hard to get a safety margin between maximal power and demands of the job. Everyone cares about the pet dog; animals need exercise for good health. Why not go out with the dog even if you don't have a dog!

PART II

GUIDELINES FOR EXERCISE PROGRAMS

INTRODUCTION

The GUIDELINES for exercise programs are principally a synthesis of opinion generated by the Symposium. In this form the relationship of one component of an exercise program to another can be more clearly seen, and their interaction can be better defined in order to prevent conflict, misunderstanding, and omission.

The *three parts* of the guidelines, "Personnel for Exercise Programs," "Program Operation," and "General Exercise Classes," are arranged in the order in which a program of exercise might be organized, but it is only a literary device, and the interaction of the parts is obvious to anyone involved in program organization. An important source of information, in addition to the formal presentation, is the ten hours of recording during the discussion sessions. Some questions arose which were not covered by the faculty in their formal presentations, and these answers are quoted below. In general, the problems discussed during these periods fell into *three categories*. One problem was the expected difficulty with communication from one specialty to another, and the following guidelines are an attempt to overcome this. A second important problem was the lack of well grounded scientific information in some fields of medical epidemiology and physiology. The third problem consisted of the limited communication which has existed between the directors of exercise programs throughout the country. It was not the purpose of this Symposium to derive a consensus of administrative solutions and technical innovations arising in highly diverse programs, but collection of this type of information no doubt represents an important objective in the future.

In general, controversy from sources outside the Symposium for "Exercise and the Heart" are avoided since it was the purpose of this Symposium and of the "Guidelines for Exercise Programs" to have the problem examined by a few well chosen people and generate an incisive opinion, not a universally inclusive one.

Chapter 12

PERSONNEL FOR EXERCISE PROGRAMS

ROBERT L. MORSE

THE necessary personnel for the execution of an exercise program has been defined by Mr. Day. Figure 12-1 represents a logical relationship between these individuals. According to the size of the exercise program various duties may be combined or expanded.

1. Exercise Program and Advisory Committee

Since the origins of exercise programs lie in enthusiasm, it would seem that a prerequisite for participation on the advisory committee would be enthusiasm for the program. However, the very existence

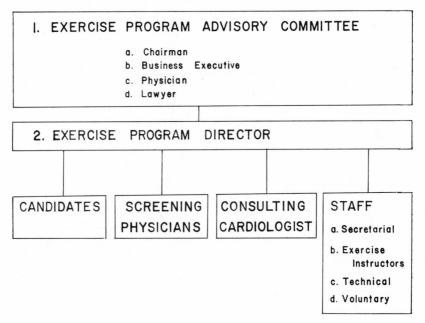

Figure 12-1

of an advisory committee, as outlined by Mr. Day, implies a responsible review of the exercise program and a check on irresponsible enthusiasm. Responsibility within the committee is delegated to at least four different members.

a. The chairman is responsible for the regular meetings held, the appointment and maintenance of the appropriate members on the committee, and an annual report.

b. An executive familiar with business practices should contribute his advice with regard to the economic status of the program, its relative priority within the framework of the whole institution, and its projected image as a public service and advertisable item. In this regard his prior experience within the exercise program should provide him with the necessary insight to evaluate and promote the exercise program with the correct soft-sell approach.

c. The physician member of the committee has three important functions. First, it is his obligation to be aware of the qualitative and quantitative features of the exercise sessions as they are being executed. He then can make a professional judgment with respect to the hazards involved in the program as well as the effectiveness of the program in accomplishing the physiologic goals which have been established. The physician would also be responsible for examination and approval of the standard physical examination form used for screening all candidates for the general exercise program. Lastly, and most difficult, is the task of finding an appropriate consulting cardiologist who can perform the very specialized function defined below with respect to the evaluation of candidates with high risk factors.

d. A member of the legal profession serving on the advisory committee could provide the specific service of establishing the form of the waiver to be used for all applicants to the exercise program. Mr. Dobrzensky outlines the form of this waiver and points out that it serves essentially to call to the attention of the applicant the fact that he assumes the ordinary risks of exercise programs. The lawyer on the advisory committee probably can serve a greater function interpreting the generalizations presented by Mr. Dobrzensky in terms of the local problems of the exercise program. While Mr. Dobrzensky mentions the use of some form of liability insurance, he stresses the preventative aspects of the legal situation. Therefore the lawyer on the advisory committee could best serve the program by defining as best as possible, the "extraordinary or unreasonable risks" that may occur in the execution of the program.

2. Program Director

Since the program director occupies a central position among all participants in the exercise program he must, in effect, be all things to all people. His capacity for leadership has been stressed by Dr. Golding and Mr. Day. His relationship to the other members of the exercise program no doubt will depend upon his personality, but several generalizations may be made about these relationships.

While his relationship with the exercise program advisory committee may be that of chief advisor and enthusiast, he is dependent upon them to serve as a cushion of authority throughout the implementation of the program. The program director's relationship to the participants is that of observer of the underlying motives of the participants, teacher of the physiology which the participant needs in order to understand the program, and counselor of the appropriate course of exercise.

The program director can help the screening physicians most by providing a concise form for the execution of the medical history and physical examination. If a consulting cardiologist with an interest in exercise can be found, he should be a great source of specific advice and information to the program director. Special examination procedures must be considered by the program director and the cardiologist together in order to manage correctly the high risk subjects with whom the cardiologist is concerned.

Other than the obvious executive relationship which the program director has with his staff, he must continually serve as a source of technical information. These duties range from physiological interpretation and formal lectures for the benefit of the program instructors to organization and guidance of a lay voluntary technical staff.

3. Candidates

Data is lacking with regard to the description of the candidates who are now participating in exercise programs. In the broadest sense they are the public, and as described by Mr. Day, can be reached by the methods of public relations, communications through the mass media, and in a more limited manner, by personal contact with previous participants in the exercise program. Dr. Golding describes a more limited population composed of sedentary people who have heard that "a sedentary existence is harmful." One program director described his population as "scared."

Clearly the population of candidates have a broad range of motivations. Since they frequently have in common the desire to improve their "fitness," Dr. Knuttgen's question "fitness for what?" is particularly useful in defining goals and possible accomplishments of the candidates. The definition of the candidates in these terms is the duty of the program director who can hopefully provide more exact information in the future.

4. Screening Physicians

The physicians who perform the screening examination for entrance into the exercise program can be the candidate's own private physician. There are at least five advantages of utilizing the candidate's personal physician for completing the medical screening test. First is the availability of such a physician. Second is the likely preference which the candidate may have in selecting a physician in whom he has confidence. Third, the examination is apt to receive more personal attention by the physician when administered to a patient with whom he is familiar. A fourth advantage of utilizing the candidate's personal physician is the subtle and entirely legitimate way in which the existence and content of the exercise program is brought to the attention of a wider range of physicians. Fifth, Mr. Dobrzensky suggests that the broader participation of physicians in the screening examinations might be advantageous in some medical-legal aspects, perhaps with respect to the contribution of a number of diverse opinions and the avoidance of a single repetitive medical opinion.

A disadvantage of utilizing the candidate's personal physician arises from his unfamiliarity with the exercise program. Many participants in the Symposium expressed their disappointment with the results of an examination conducted by physicians who understood little about the objectives of the program and seemed too willing to provide a blanket endorsement of an exercise program. In this case it seems that a brief description of the exercise program and some of its pertinent physiology could be provided to the physician along with the examination form. In this case the physician is more likely to render a thoughtful opinion based upon the pertinent facts of the case.

5. Consulting Cardiologist

An expert opinion in physiological and medical matters is most likely to be available to the program in the form of a consulting cardiologist, although it was suggested that such personnel could be found in the fields of physical medicine, rehabilitation, and preventative medicine. It was emphasized that this cardiologist be especially aware of the problems related to exercise programs, since general opinions from otherwise well qualified specialists have been disappointing and sometimes have been described as untrustworthy. These special opinions are most likely to be concerned with the initiation of the program and possibly could be supplied on a consultation basis by a visiting group of specialists from an academic community. However, this solution to the supply problem of specialized expert opinion does not answer the question in two cases. The first case is the recurrent problem of candidates with high risk factors as described by Dr. Kannel. A cardiologist familiar with both the risk factors and the therapeutic possibilities of exercise is needed to render an appropriate opinion on such candidates. An even more ambitious question is that of exercise programs for candidates with known cardiac disease. Such a cardiologist is necessary here also.

6. Staff

A secretarial staff is essential for the smooth and consistent operation of the exercise program, especially for the processing of the candidate applications. In addition, the follow-up of physiologic status and attendance status by secretarial help can contribute greatly to the integrity of the program. Lastly, of great importance in the future will be the long-term follow-up of participants in exercise programs, a procedure which can not be accomplished without a secretarial staff.

The most important staff is the actual exercise class instructor, one of whom could be the program director himself. As Dr. Golding clearly describes, the personal characteristics of the class instructors are most important in leading the class to its goal of physical conditioning.

Mr. Day emphasizes the use of lay personnel in assisting the execution of the exercise program. The most obvious use of such personnel is with physiological testing, secretarial duties, public relations, and exercise class leaders or assistant leaders.

Chapter 13

PROGRAM OPERATION

ROBERT L. MORSE

A FLOW chart of candidates proceeding from the initial interview to completion of the exercise program is presented in Figure 13-1. The status of each candidate can thus be defined, and his future progress can be clearly outlined.

1. Initial Interview

If long-term benefit to the patient as well as long-term effectiveness of the program is important, a critical juncture of the program is the initial interview between the candidates and the program director. Likely the candidate has decided to give the program a try, but equally likely he has no definite idea about a long-term commitment. It is the duty of the program director to help the candidate be specific as to what he could try to accomplish with an exercise program. The director therefore will have to fathom the candidate's motives and classify them into various categories. His motives might be the following: a return to previous states of agility, strength, and endurance; a cosmetic improvement; a desire to join a special group, or a desire merely to "do something" for fear of aging. Difficult to define, but perhaps best described by Dr. Chapman as a "tranquilizing effect," exercise may be desired mostly for its psychological benefits.

At this point the program director must become an instructor of physiology. However this instruction is accomplished, whether during the initial interview, in formal lectures, or in multiple sessions prior to each exercise class, the program director and the class instructors need to cover the basic physiology described by Drs. Rowell, Åstrand, and Knuttgen. Special emphasis should be given to the differentiation between exercise programs for improving muscular strength, programs for developing skills, and programs for improving

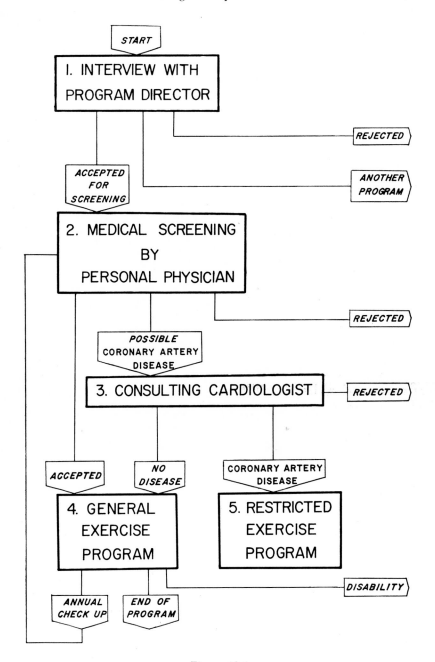

Figure 13-1

aerobic power. The various components of the program which contain these three factors obviously will have more meaning and be of greater interest to the candidate once he appreciates their difference. This Symposium was, of course, most concerned with cardiac responses largely measured by evaluations of aerobic power. Therefore, the emphasis here is upon those procedures that influence and test cardiac performance and oxygen consumption. Drs. Knuttgen and Åstrand stress these tests both in their formal presentation and in the summary discussions.

After the initial interview the program director has three options, as illustrated by Figure 13-1. Candidates should be rejected from further consideration if they do not have the motivation to see them through one cycle of the program. A second option of the program director is an exact exercise recommendation concerning activity which is specifically suited to the objectives of the candidate. If impressive biceps are what the candidate needs, then a jogging program will be disappointing and useless. If it is his game of tennis or golf which concerns him most, then clearly he should be directed to a professional instructor of such skills. Another example of a specialized program is that of the lone jogger or the lone exerciser. This type of exercise as described by Dr. Åstrand may be the most common in the world. In any case, medical screening prior to these other programs is recommended. If little statistical information is available about organized exercise programs, virtually none is available about the average lone exerciser. While this subject obviously merits great emphasis, the present Symposium was not designed for its extensive coverage.

The third option is that of accepting the candidate for the exercise program, at which point he is referred to his personal physician for medical screening.

2. Medical Screening by Personal Physician

The medical screening can be done by the candidate's personal physician. It will be greatly facilitated by providing the physician with a simple examination form and a description of the exercise program. Several features contribute to the effectiveness of the examination form. First, the basic questions of medical history could be stated in a "yes" or "no" manner, so that most of the history could be completed by the candidate before seeing his physician. Secondly, certain laboratory values could be obtained prior to the physician's examination. For instance, measurements described by Dr. Kannel, such as skin fold, weight, girth, and flexibility, could be obtained at the time of the initial interview. More specific medical testing, such as vital capacity, forced expiratory flow rate, electrocardiogram, chest x-ray, and standard blood tests, could also be obtained prior to the examination, provided that these examinations were ordered under the supervision of a physician and performed by competent technical personnel. Otherwise, these examinations are best left to the personal physician to arrange.

Appendix A contains an outline of a possible screening examination at the end of which the physician is lead to one of four opinions. Three of these opinions, namely advising a general exercise program, advising a special exercise program, or advising against an exercise program, are straightforward. However, abnormalities of history, physical examination, or laboratory data, which prevent outright approval or disapproval of exercise, raise problems. As Drs. Kannel and Åstrand have pointed out, the abnormalities of the screening examination which leads one to be cautious about an exercise program may in fact be the most important reasons for entering the candidate into an exercise program.

While there are no established guidelines for the handling of these borderline individuals, Dr. Kannel is willing to give us an opinion. He suggests that the exercise electrocardiogram (which would be done if the resting electrocardiogram were normal) be one arbitrator of the question of whether the candidate should be placed in a restricted or in a general exercise program. The candidates who would be tested by exercise electrocardiograms would be anyone who exhibited a blood pressure over 160/95, a cholesterol above 260, a blood sugar taken two hours after a meal of above 160, or those with excessive obesity or exhibiting breathlessness on a standard exercise test which raises the heart beyond a reasonable target value. In addition, Dr. Kannel suggested placing those candidates who exhibit any two of the above abnormalities in a restricted exercise program anyway.

This scheme implies the capability of performing exercise electrocardiograms as well as the availability of a restricted exercise program for cardiac patients and those candidates with high risk factors. Such a test and such a program is best conducted by a cardiologist whose consultation implements the time-honored practice of obtaining a second opinion in cases of doubtful disposition.

Is the entire medical examination necessary for young subjects? The answer is that a full medical investigation as described above is probably not always necessary, and below the age of thirty-five, the basic history and physical examination, if normal, are adequate. In those over thirty-five, however it seems that the additional examination of blood tests and resting electrocardiogram are indicated. This advice would apply to all types of exercise programs, whether team competition, lone jogging, or YMCA exercise classes.

3. *Consulting Cardiologist*

A consulting cardiologist is the only consultant described in these guidelines because his task is most pertinent to the purposes of the Symposium. The screening physician might well want other consultations—orthopedic, endocrinological, etc., whose opinions are well defined and present fewer problems to the administration of the exercise program.

In general, the cardiologist wishes to diagnose illnesses which might contraindicate a general exercise program, the foremost illness being significant and unstable coronary artery disease. The suspicion of occult coronary artery disease is raised by the presence of nonspecific risk factors, such as the subject's age, sex, abnormalities of physical examination, blood pressure, serum cholesterol, and smoking habits. Such findings as nonspecific electrocardiographic abnormalties still do not prove the presence of the disease although he might make a presumptive diagnosis at this time which would be valid for the purpose of the exercise program.

In addition to re-evaluating the data collected by the referring physician, he can proceed to one of two definitive tests of coronary artery disease. These tests are the exercise electrocardiogram and the coronary arteriogram. Suffice it to say that the latter requires hospitalization and is used only for diagnosis in special clinical situations and for consideration of surgical treatment of coronary artery disease.

The exercise electrocardiogram is the most important test beyond the standard history, physical examination, and laboratory tests.

The subject of exercise electrocardiography was not emphasized in this Symposium and is a subject of wide interest and study. Many reviews of this subject are available* A few general statements might be made here. The technique of the exercise electrocardiogram is the prerogative of the cardiologist since there is no universally acceptable technique at the present time. The principal differences between one method and another consist of the amount of exercise and the type of ECG lead. The amount of exercise is important since the yield of positive cases increases with higher levels of exercise. The amount of exercise which has been used varies from relatively low levels established by the Master's Test to those of maximal exercise levels utilizing a treadmill or a bicycle ergometer. It was suggested in the question-and-answer period that the candidates should be tested with exercise to workloads experienced in the program itself. A better plan is testing the candidates with increasing workloads until a "target" heart rate is achieved. Such a plan is outlined in more detail in the following section, "General Exercise Classes."

Having repeated the history and physical examination, and having surveyed the laboratory data, resting ECG, and exercise ECG (if done), the cardiologist can recommend one of three courses of action as outlined in Figure 13-1. Exercise may be contraindicated because of congestive heart failure, hypertension, peripheral vascular disease, documented exercise-induced arrhythmias, etc. It is likely this group of patients should be on some form of therapy and in some cases may be re-evaluated for an exercise program at a later date.

At the opposite end of the spectrum are the patients with some risk factor abnormality but negative exercise electrocardiograms. These subjects may be the best candidates for the therapeutic possibilities of an exercise program. The rest of the candidates have documented or great likelihood of coronary artery disease and should not be allowed in a general exercise program. Exercise may be of great value to them but their exercise program must be specially designed and monitored. The burden of establishing and executing such

---

*One such review: Blackburn, Henry: *Measurements in Exercise Electrocardiography.* Springfield, Thomas, 1969..

a program would lie with the consulting cardiologist himself and represents an extensive investment of his own time and energy as described by Dr. Hirsch.

4. General Exercise Classes

The general exercise classes and their integral component, the physiologic testing, are designed to accept the general population who has no contraindication for such exercise. They are described in greater detail in Chapter 14. While occupying a central position as defined by Figure 13-1, the exercise classes are merely one station in the execution of the whole program. Furthermore in a larger sense the whole program is in turn one station in the whole life of the candidate. So when all is said and done what difference has this little experience of the exercise classes made to the candidate? The time to review this question is when the candidate exits from the exercise classes and re-cycles through an annual checkup or to the program director prior to leaving the program.

In the first place the program should have been pleasant—hopefully, pleasurable. If the candidate started dreading exercise, the program must have taught him that it need not be dreadful. If the candidate started optimistically, the atmosphere of the program should have been conservative enough to avoid an anticlimax. A group exercise program offers great advantages in presenting exercise in a friendly, perhaps convivial, environment. Here everyone has been reduced (or elevated) to the same common basis of activity and accomplishment, and the participant's experience may be more impressive and memorable when compared to the rest of the group.

In the second place, the exercise classes should have made a subjective and objective change in his physical condition which is perfectly evident to him. Clearly, the program must be at least this powerful. This, however, may not be very long lasting, since, as Dr. Åstrand pointed out, complete deconditioning can occur within one month and muscular atrophy can occur much faster in complete inactivity.

The long-term results of the program must be of subtle educational nature which in turn can lead to a change in long-term exercise habits. It is really more important (and obviously easier) if the exercise leader advises rather than directs. The candidate can take over the conduct of his program before he leaves, and he can reproduce its effects elsewhere and on his own. His exercise is clearly his business, and he has to take the responsibility for it. He must become an expert with regard to his own physical condition since there are few others around him who can substitute.

5. Restricted Exercise Classes

Exercise programs for patients with known or suspected coronary artery disease are distinctly different from exercise programs for the general population. As Drs. Kannel and Hirsch carefully outlined, these programs are restricted in terms of selected subjects with high risk factors and also restricted in terms of the amount and types of exercise which these subjects are encouraged to perform.

Everyone, including the participants of the Symposium, agreed these programs must be separate from the general exercise programs. They were obviously of great interest, first of all, because they apparently are feasible. From Dr. Hirsch's data, which is authoritative in this field, exercise programs designed for cardiac patients do not seem to be particularly dangerous. On the contrary, at the present time it seems a possibility that such programs are of benefit to the patients, at least in terms of psychological and physiological parameters. Such benefits, if achieved with low risk, are very worthwhile to the practice of medicine. An important question however, that of the possible benefit to morbidity and mortality, has yet to be answered, and such data is not clearly forthcoming soon.

Despite the general agreement that cardiac patients should not be included in general exercise programs, there still recurs the question of why some of these patients, who have no detectable functional defects, should not be allowed in these general programs. Mr. Dobrzensky touches on this subject when he suggests that a responsible institution offering an intelligent exercise program is obviously providing a service of implied quality. The participants in such a program would have a right to expect this quality, part of which would be its safety. It seems that in return, the institution has the right and the responsibility to err on the conservative side in excluding those candidates who have a known high risk of sudden death or a myocardial infarction which might be attributed to the exercise program.

There are a number of special considerations which differentiate the restricted exercise program from the general exercise program. First of all the careful examination of a cardiologist with the special interest described above is necessary. Not only are the appropriate screening examinations needed, but special attention to evidence of congestive heart failure, paroxysmal hypertension, cardiac arrhythmias, or unstable coronary artery disease is necessary. Furthermore, such evaluations must necessarily be repeated at regular intervals as described by Dr. Hirsch.

The necessity for exercise testing is obvious, and its results would be important factors in the consideration of the prescription of exercise. The exercise prescription, that is, the *amount* and *type* of exercise which is recommended, must be established for every subject and must be more specific than that utilized in the general exercise program. Follow-up interview and review of the subject performance during the exercise program is necessary for progressive change in the prescription.

The execution of the exercise classes might follow the general exercise programs and could be conducted by the same exercise instructor. However, with this group of patients it seems reasonable that there be immediate access to trained medical personnel who could accomplish expert resuscitation. Such equipment, as a cardiac defribillator, laryngoscope, endotracheal tube, intravenous tubing and fluids, and various emergency drugs, must all be available. Such a program amounts to a considerable medical operation, but the future may well prove that it need not be a prohibitive enterprise for many institutions interested in such a program.

Chapter 14

GENERAL EXERCISE CLASSES

ROBERT L. MORSE

GENERAL exercise classes are meant to accomodate the general population and provide a general selection of exercises with its program. The principal components of general classes as illustrated in Figure 14-1 are objective measurements, subjective symptom check, and exercise classes.

1. Objective Testing

While objective testing usually implies the measurement of some physiologic variable, such as heart rate, duration of time taken to run a certain distance, the subject's weight, etc., other types of observations are clearly useful, such as obesity, shortness of breath, gait disturbance, etc. In general there are four reasons for physiologic testing: for motivational purposes, for placement of subjects in high or low exercise groups, for measurements of training effects on the participants, and for the evaluation of the exercise program itself and comparison of it with others.

When used for motivational purposes, the tests must be understood by the participant so he can derive satisfaction from the result. The educational nature of the instructor's job is evident here.

When used for placement in high or low exercise groups, testing and measuring may simply consist of an experienced eye cast upon a corpulent and dyspneic candidate, or may more elaborately consist of a measurement of aerobic power.

When objective testing is used as a measurement of the physiologic changes produced by the exercise program, one must be as precise as possible about defining what physiology needs measuring. If the purpose of the program is for the candidate to reduce his weight, then obviously weighing him is the single most important measurement

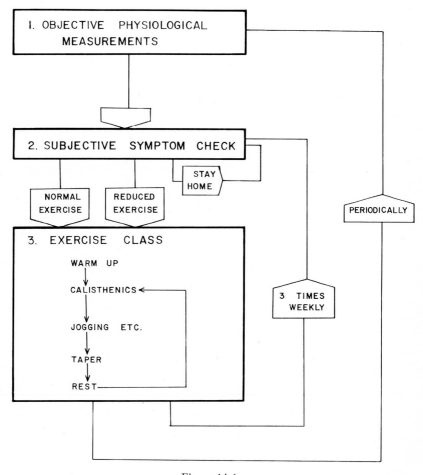

Figure 14-1.

Likewise, if the size of the biceps is important, then a tape measure is all that is necessary. If aerobic power is of interest, then the equipment necessary to measure it must be obtained.

The use of physiologic testing for the purpose of comparing one exercise program with another leads immediately to a scientific inquiry as to the best techniques of measuring as well as the best techniques of exercise. The program staff will be exposed to the details of exercise physiology and in turn will be better equipped to evaluate and criticize their own program. In this way the physiologic testing is a link between the practical program and the scientific world from which new developments with important implications are likely to come.

Of prime interest to the Symposium is the measurement of cardiac function. In normal individuals it is the heart which determines the limits of exercise, and reciprocally it is exercise which can be used to measure the limits of cardiac function.

TABLE 14-I

HYPOTHETICAL VALUES OF PHYSOLOGIC PARAMETERS DURING EXERCISE IN FIFTY-YEAR-OLD ABNORMAL, NORMAL, AND CONDITIONED SUBJECTS

	Abnormal	*Normal*	*Conditioned*
Oxygen Consumption (milliliters per minute)			
Rest	250	250	250
Mild stress	510	730	1070
Moderate stress	790	1070	1490
"Target" stress	1070	1420	1900
Maximal stress	1640	2100	2720
Heart Rate (beats per minute)			
Rest	82	72	60
Mild stress	100	100	100
Moderate stress	120	120	120
"Target" stress	140	140	140
Maximal stress	180	180	180
Stroke Volume (milliliters)			
Rest	58	74	89
Mild stress	58	74	89
Moderate stress	58	74	89
"Target" stress	58	74	89
Maximal stress	58	74	89
Cardiac Output (liters per minute)			
Rest	4.8	5.3	5.3
Mild stress	5.8	7.4	8.9
Moderate stress	7.0	8.9	10.6
"Target" stress	8.1	10.4	12.4
Maximal stress	10.4	13.3	16.0
Arteriovenous Oxygen Difference (volume percentage)			
Rest	5.3	4.7	4.7
Mild stress	8.7	9.8	12.1
Moderate stress	11.3	12.1	14.0
"Target" stress	13.2	13.7	15.3
Maximal stress	15.8	15.8	17.0

Table 14-I,* presenting hypothetical physiological values, has been constructed to condense eight principles if exercise testing and physiology covered in detail by Åstrand, Rowell, and Knuttgen.

a. Maximum heart rate is predicted for each individual according to his age. Åstrand quotes values which are approximated by subtracting the age of the individual from 220. He points out that this prediction may not be very precise, and it may be wrong by fifteen beats per minute.

b. Target heart rate is selected as the highest heart rate at which individuals will be exercised. It is usually calculated as some percentage of the maximal heart rate. In Table 14-I it is 78 percent. Åstrand quotes target heart rates which are approximated by subtracting the age of the individual from 195. This results in about 85 percent of maximal heart rate.

c. The immediate response of the heart to any single bout of exercise is principally a change in heart rate. Whatever stroke volume is present at rest remains approximately the same throughout the bout of exercise.

d. The long-term response of the heart to repeated bouts of exercise during conditioning is an increase in resting stroke volume. Of course, as above, each bout of exercise is accompanied by an increase in heart rate, but the conditioned individual starts off with, and maintains, a higher stroke volume.

e. The resting heart rate will be lower in conditioned individuals. This is because an individual needs the same cardiac output at rest whether conditioned or not. Therefore, if he has a higher stroke volume, the heart rate at rest will be appropriately lower.

f. Stress is best measured by the individual's heart rate response, although shortness of breath, fatigue, and pain are obviously important. In Table 14-I, for instance, moderate stress is a heart rate of 120 regardless of the condition of the individual.

g. The oxygen consumption at any given stress is different from one individual to another according to his conditioning. Conversely, the same oxygen consumption, such as 1070 in Table 14-I, repre-

---

*Table 14-I presents values which are obtained from the Fick equation explained by Rowell and are constrained by the assumption that stroke volume is constant during a single bout of exercise.

sents a different stress to different individuals. It also results in different physiological reactions as the other underlined values reveal.

h. The best practical test of cardiovascular conditioning is the measurement of external work production on a bicycle ergometer during exercise stress. The amount of stress, that is the "target stress," is adjusted to achieve some percentage of maximal heart rate. External work production can be converted into oxygen consumption by Åstrand's Figure 2-16. In order to compare one individual with another the work rate or oxygen consumption should be divided by the body mass.

Maximal stress testing is the only reliable method of measuring aerobic power, but should *not* be performed in any but controlled laboratory conditions. Aerobic power might be approximated by linear extrapolation from sub-maximal exercise data, as Table 14-1 illustrates.[*]

The blood pressure represents an important measure of cardiac physiology. Since it is known that average blood pressure rises little in the normal person during exercise, inappropriately high blood pressures during exercise is an important pathological observation and may represent significant disability to patients with cardiac disease. Plethysmography, ballistocardiography, and peripheral pulse recordings are of interest in certain research situations and can reliably reflect heart rate. But these devices, some of which are presently used in fitness programs, cannot measure the force of cardiac contraction, which is more properly defined as "contractility." Measurements of contractility at the present time require elaborate laboratory equipment unavailable to the usual exercise program.

2. Subjective Symptom Check

It is common sense that exercise classes should be discontinued in the presence of acute illness. In a program of well adults it is clearly up to the participant whether he feels well and should exercise. How should he be guided with regard to the frequent states between obvious illness and obvious well-being? A few generalizations could be stated here, although specific application must always be individualized.

a. Cardiovascular illness. Chest pain or pressure, palpitations, fainting, light-headedness, irregular pulse and shortness of breath are the principle symptoms of heart disease, and these should contraindicate exercise and indicate medical examination.

b. Respiratory illnesses. A mild upper respiratory illness need not be a contraindication to exercise, but fever, pharyngitis, aggravated by breathing, a productive cough, or wheezing should be contraindications. A common respiratory illness is smoking.

c. Gastrointestinal illness. A recent heavy meal alone is a contraindication to exercise. Abdominal distress of mild degree may represent functional or infectious illness which would not contraindicate exercise, but in combination with fever, tachycardia, nausea, vomiting, or diarrhea, such distress is a contraindication. The participants with known gastrointestinal diseases, gall bladder disease, ulcer disease, diverticulitis, hemorrhoids, etc. need the advice of their own physician as to how much symptomatology (if any) is to be permitted.

d. Orthopedic disease. Dr. Hamrell described orthopedic illnesses which have been seen in exercise classes. Acute swelling, tenderness, or pain of any significant magnitude is a contraindication to exercise. A physician's advice is necessary before continuing with an orthopedic illness except for minor aches and pains.

Some of the above illnesses may lead to a physician's "checkup" and further medical screening. As indicated in Figure 14-1, the results of such an examination may lead to rejection from the program, a different program of exercise, or eventual return to the original program.

Although not a disease, an important subjective symptom to check is the reaction to ambient temperature and humidity. As Dr. Knuttgen points out, the program director should be aware of the problem and limit the class appropriately. At the same time the participants should learn the limits for their own good.

As described by some participants in the Symposium, some programs have a "buddy system" of checking on subjective complaints prior to each exercise class. This may be useful in relieving the individual of some of his embarrassment of admitting to an illness about which he is reluctant to volunteer information. It may also help adherence to the program.

The results of these symptom-checks may be the decision to refrain from exercise; likely, the participant merely decides to stay home. Another result of the symptom check might be the decision to restrict temporarily the level of his exercise for a single exercise session. In this case he could take advantage of the built-in flexibility described by Dr. Hirsch which an exercise class must have. In this way he can place himself in a lower group temporarily.

3. Exercise Class

Dr. Golding wishes to avoid a specific answer to the question "What exercises should be done in an exercise program?" because the best exercises are a function of the local variables; the physical plant, the experience of the program director, and the various preferences of the participants. However, Dr. Golding is specific about certain categories of exercise and the sequence in which they might be used.

a. Warm-up is clearly necessary before any extensive exercise, although the exact reason for this has not clearly been established. It seems likely that it accomplishes "musculoskeletal preconditioning;" that is, stretching of the muscles, flexing and extending of joints, and testing of principal skills and postures to be used later in the exercise session. Dr. Åstrand mentioned the beneficial changes within joint spaces and joint cartilages induced by the initial exercise.

Perhaps most important is the initial and gradual activation of cardiovascular mechanisms, such as blood volume shifts induced by vasodilitation of the lungs, skin, and muscles and by visceral vasoconstriction. Tachycardia at this time should not be excessive, and when properly accomplished, warm-up should prevent sudden stepwise changes in blood pressure or peripheral resistance.

b. Calisthenics, muscular strengthening, skill development, or competitive activities all have in common the accomplishment of specific goals and not necessarily that of cardiovascular conditioning. This type of activity may well represent the goals of the participant and obviously has to be developed individually by each program. It is obviously valuable in maintaining motivation and interest in the program. Carried to its extremes, however, the members of the Symposium agreed that this type of activity usually carried a high risk of musculoskeletal injury and undesirable peaks of cardiovascular stress in unconditioned participants.

c. Cardiovascular conditioning occupies the main focus of the exercise programs as concerned in this Symposium. It is accomplished by large muscle group exercises, jogging, bicycle riding, swimming, etc. It needs to be carried to an intensity resulting in a "target" tachycardia which is determined principally by the subject's age, as outlined in the previous section on testing. Dr. Åstrand outlines a minimal exercise program which lasts for one-half hour and is repeated at least three times weekly.

It is obvious that the level of exercise early in the program should be low, perhaps only walking in older age groups. The advantage of an organized exercise program is the guidance of the exercise instructors who can provide for gradual, overall increase in the exercise level, as well as a simultaneous variety of levels within the class.

While target heart rate seems to be a good criteria of the level of the exercise to be chosen, Dr. Åstrand mentions several practical points, such as limiting exercise to the level which one can still speak comfortably and, in general, limiting exercise to what is comfortable to the rest of the body. Discomfort would also limit exercise in the presence of high temperature and high humidity.

d. Tapering exercises are especially important after higher levels of exercise. The redistribution of blood volume accomplished by exercise is of principal interest here, and tapering exercise prevents untoward peripheral pooling of blood which can result in postural hypotension and fainting. A different reason for tapering may be a beneficial effect upon the cardiac rhythm. Tapering implements the general rule of avoiding sudden step-wise changes in activity.

Another postexercise rule raised by several participants of the Symposium is that of avoiding hot showers immediately after exercise. Likely peripheral pooling of blood volume is again the problem in this case although more severe toxicity has been reported as described in Dr. Lown's discussion. A cold environment, that is a cool shower, seems to have no significant adverse effect.

The end of an exercise program is either a seasonal event defined by the program director or a personal decision by the participant. However, it is clear that there is no abrupt end of exercise, and the details of what happens to the participant's conditioning may be the most important epidemiological question of such programs. Information here would clearly have a most profound influence upon guidelines of future exercise programs.

APPENDIX A

HISTORY AND PHYSICAL EXAMINATION

Name_____

Date _____ Age _____.

1. GENERAL MEDICAL HISTORY

Any medical complaints? _____Yes_____ No_____

Any major illnesses in the past? (Give dates.)_____Yes_____ No_____

Any hospitalization? _____Yes_____ No_____

Smoke now?_____ Packages per day _____

Smoked in past?_____ Packages per day _____

Weight gain in past ten years _____

Weight at age 20_____ 30_____ 40_____ 50_____

Diabetes? Yes_____ No_____ Family history of diabetes. Who?_____

Family history of heart disease. Who?_____

Family history of high blood pressure. Who?_____

Family history of muscular illness. Who?_____

2. CARDIORESPIRATORY HISTORY

Any heart disease now? Yes__ No__   High blood pressure?   Yes__ No__

Shortness of breath at

Any heart disease in   rest?   Yes__ No__

past?   Yes__ No__   Shortness of breath

Heart murmurs   Yes__ No__   supine?   Yes__ No__

Occasional chest pains? Yes__ No__   Shortness of breath after

Chest pains on exertion? Yes__ No__   one flight of stairs? Yes__ No__

Palpitation?   Yes__ No__   Daily coughing?   Yes__ No__

Fainting?   Yes__ No__   Cough produces sputum?

Yes__ No__

3. MUSCULAR HISTORY

Any muscle injuries or   Muscular illness now? Yes__ No__

illnesses now?   Yes__ No__   Muscle pain at rest? Yes__ No__

Any muscle injuries or   Muscle pains on exertion?

illnesses in past? Yes__ No__   Yes__ No__

Muscle weakness now? Yes__ No__

4. BONE—JOINT HISTORY

Any bone or joint (including spine) Flat feet?   Yes__ No__

injuries or illnesses   Athletics in past?   Yes__ No__

now.?   Yes__ No__   Specify _____

Any bone or joint (in-
cluding spine) injury
or illnesses in past? Yes__ No__

Ever have swollen joints? Yes__ No__
Ever have painful joints? Yes__ No__

5. LABORATORY EXAMINATION

Height _____ Weight _____ Girth _____
Fat thickness, arm _____ Scapula _____
Vital capacity _____ Forced expiratory volume (1 second)_____
ECG Rate _____ Rhythm _____ Axis _____
Interpretation _____
BLOOD—Hematocrit_____ Hemoglobin_____ White Cell Count_____
      Cholesterol (fasting)_____ Blood Sugar (2 hrs after meal)_____
URINALYSIS—Special Gravity_____ Protein_____ Sugar_____
CHEST X-RAY—Interpretation _____

6 PHYSICAL EXAMINATION

Thyroid abnormal?	Yes__ No__	Peripheral pulses
Chest auscultation		absent? Yes__ No__
Abnormal?	Yes__ No__	Any joints abnormal? Yes__ No__
Heart size abnormal?	Yes__ No__	Abdominal masses? Yes__ No__
Murmurs present?	Yes__ No__	Hernia? Yes__ No__
Gallops, abnormal		Blood pressure_____
heart sounds?	Yes__ No__	Pulse rate_____

SUMMARY IMPRESSION OF PHYSICIAN

1. Comments of any history or physical finding (especially "yes" answers):_____
_____

Diagnoses: _____

2. Opinion (Select one)
   (a) Participation in a moderately vigorous exercise program is advisable,
   and there is no contraindication evident by this examination
   (b) Participation in exercise other than a general exercise program, namely
   _____, is advisable, and there is no con-
   traindication evident by this examination.
   (c) Participation in a moderately vigorous general exercise program *may be
   advisable,* but before such a program is instituted, further examination
   or consultation is necessary, namely_____
   (d) Because of the above diagnosis, participation in a moderately vigorous
   general exercise program is *inadvisable.*
               Signed_____M.D.

RELEASE

I hereby release the above information to the exercise program director.
            Signed_____

INDEX

A

Acetylene method, measuring cardiac output, xiv
Adenosine triphosphate, 225
Adipose tissue biopsy, 145
Adult education program, 70
Advisory committee, 230, 231
Aerobic and anerobic processes, 27-28, 29
Aerobic capacity, 54, 59-60, 61
Aerobic energy yield, 27
Aerobic muscular activity, 55
Aerobic power, 214, 237, 245, 246, 249
Aerobic power and performance, 34
Aerobic power, maximal, 29, 36
  factors for increase, 42
Aerobics program, 67
Age adjustment, 155
Agility, 68
Air temperature
  dry bulb, 58
  wet bulb, 58
Alactacid Oxygen debt, 29
Alexander, John F., 199
Ambient conditions, 57
Ambient temperature and humidity, 250
Ambient water vapor tension, 58
American Heart Association, 128, 169
Anaerobic capacity, maximal, 29
Anaerobic energy yield, 27, 46
Anaerobic processes, 29
Anemia, severe, 84, 91
Aneurysms, 203
Angina pectoris, 108, 110, 113, 114, 115, 121, 123, 134, 135, 143, 144, 159, 172, 200, 201, 203, 204 208, 220, 221
  and exercise conditioning, 200
Angiograms, 130
Ankle edema, 113

Antiarrhythmic drugs, 152
Anthropometrical measurements, 68
Arbaquez, 115
Argument to the jury, 103
Arrhythmias, 107, 126, 152, 154, 201, 203, 204, 208, 209
Arterial enzymes, 131
Arterial lactate response, 134
Arterial pressure, 22, 121
Arterial pulses, 113
Arterioles responses, 16
ASHD, 107, 109, 110, 111, 115, 117, 122, 125, 127, 128, 129, 131, 132, 133, 134, 139, 146, 150, 151, 152, 159, 160, 162, 163, 165, 166, 167, 168, 170, 172,
  and prohibited practices, 162-63,
  regimen
    physical training, 109
    risk factors, 109
  vs. NCP, 108
Åstrand, Per-Olof, 27, 115, 213, 236, 238, 239, 242, 248, 249, 251, 252
Asymptomatic, 140, 159, 171
  subjects, 122, 125, 129
Atherogenic traits, 88, 219
Atherosclerosis, 82, 88,
  and treatment, 169
Atherosclerotic heart disease (ASHD), and therapeutic value of physical conditioning, 107
Atherosclerotic lesions, 108
Atherothrombotic stenosis, 83
Athlete's heart superiority, 82
ATP, 28-29
Atrial and ventricular depolarization. 155
Atrial temperature, 22
Atrioventricular conduction defects. 159
A-V Oxygen difference, 6, 12, 13, 15, 16, 19, 41-42, 247